Songs

That

Remember

By Carol Oen

ISBN 978-0-9840015-0-7

Author Contact:
    write4you2read@gmail.com

Published by ^{The}One_{Company}

Acknowledgments

It takes a village to write a book. Thoughtful, insightful, intelligent, well-read and well-written individuals populate my necessary village.

Barbara Barrett
Deirdre Barrett
Barbara and Phil Brady
Woody and Ruth Gove
Merry Ann Hansen
Les and Frankie Hulett
Annie Long
Elizabeth and Joshua Mitchell
Robert Nelson
Dean Oen
John Oen
Helen Randolph
Mona Raridon and her writers' group: Jane Flanagan, Roz Gift, Elsie Knoke, and Margaret Pennycook
Ann Stanley
Ethel Steinhauer
Elizabeth Stone
Kristin Stone
Iris Swift
Jane Williams

Friends who have shared their experiences with Alzheimer's-afflicted loved ones.

1 Jack

Marsha Rutherford sat clutching the arms of her wheelchair as though she couldn't let go. She looked like a small bird, perched on her hands, mouth open. Jack patiently pushed the last spoonful of oatmeal into his wife's mouth. Swallowing had moved up on the long list of her problems.

"Marsha, you did great with your breakfast! I know you were hungry, Sweetheart. That's a good girl." Jack wiped her face with a napkin, then she sat quietly in her wheelchair twisting her fingers in different patterns, watching them as though she'd never seen these hands before. Marsha had retreated into herself, where she stayed almost all the time.

Jack stacked their two trays and empty food containers and shoved them to the far end of the table, out of their way. There would be some time before Marsha's next appointment and this large cafeteria interested him. He sat back to relax and watch other people.

Here he was, at The Clinic some called America's Medical Mecca. Kind of exciting to be here. He felt a twinge of guilt, wishing he'd brought Marsha years ago when it might have made a difference in the progression of her Alzheimer's disease.

The cafeteria lay tucked below ground, many stories under the top of the building. A large glass and metal dome over one corner of the room provided a glimpse of sky and if you looked way up, you could see nearby tall buildings. Cafeteria tables clustered around huge white columns. Smells of toasted bread and coffee identified morning.

At first sight of The Clinic, he'd been captivated by the clean, neat, architecturally interesting exterior. Down here the wide swath of people caught his interest and his imagination. Perhaps most were patients with family members; some might be employees having their breakfasts.

Tables seated two, four, or eight persons. Most seemed to be for four, like theirs. Many had chairless spaces to accommodate wheelchairs. No canned music, just the steady hum arising from a crowd of talking people. The conversing choir melded with intricate rhythms of moving feet and food.

This Monday morning looked busy, with most tables filled. Perhaps all mornings exhibited the same traffic. He wondered.

They'd been up extra early to be here by 7:00, ready for lab tests. Marsha fasted before her blood draw, so the cafeteria beckoned after that. It seemed better to pass the spare time here than wandering around the buildings.

Many people coming in, but few leaving—all ages from babies in strollers to folks who looked like centenarians, some looking vigorous, others obviously ill, some moving purposefully, and others haltingly. Some wore garb suggesting they came from exotic, far-away places and some looked like local farmers with rough skin tanned deeply up to a hat line topped by very pale foreheads.

So many wheelchairs. Clearly a place for the infirm. At the street-level entrance, rows of empty wheelchairs awaited patients who would like to use them. He had brought Marsha's along in the plane from California. Well, maybe she'd need it later.

"Are these seats taken?" A blond woman wearing dark green slacks and a bright green shirt pushed a man in a wheelchair up to the table. Jack guessed they were mid-60s to mid-70s, about the same ages as he and Marsha.

"They're available," Jack gestured to the seats. He smiled, but couldn't think of anything else to say. To himself he said, "God, my social skills are dormant. This isn't like me." He said nothing more.

The woman busied herself settling the man into the space and locking his chair's wheels. She left to retrieve two trays, one with oatmeal, a cardboard container of milk, and toast. This she set before the man. The other she set down at the place next to him. That held an omelet, toast and coffee. Still standing, she opened the milk container for him and then turned to arrange her own tray.

Jack's eye caught a sudden movement across from Marsha. The man pulled his tray off the table, turned it up, and shoved it down along his body, plopping breakfast contents hither and thither on their way to the floor, where they settled into islands surrounded by milk. The tray skittered under Marsha and stopped.

"No, oh please, please no. No more…" Across the table Jack watched as the dark green, then the light green of clothing sank, dropping from an upright line to completely disappear. The man then reached for the woman's tray, but Jack managed to grab it and move it out of his reach.

Jack waited a full minute, but the woman didn't reappear. He bent down to check the floor-level activity. She was crumpled on her knees, head down, hands over her face, shoulders heaving with muffled sobs.

He didn't know how far the food thrower could reach, so Jack quickly scanned the table to see if there was anything else that needed to be moved away from him. Then he got down on all fours to approach the crying woman.

Moving awkwardly to her side, his knee arthritis protested. He stretched out an arm over the woman's shoulders, saying gently, "There, there, it's OK. Everything will be OK. No harm done."

She continued weeping in her crouched position. Jack laboriously scooted around to face her. Darned awkward maneuvering under a cafeteria table, he thought. From this position, he reached for her hands, continuing to mumble words he hoped would be soothing. Then he pulled her toward him.

She put her head on his shoulder, and he held her, continuing to talk, trying to reassure her that the world hadn't come to an end as he massaged her back. Over a few minutes she gradually stopped crying, but hung on to him as though she were in danger of drowning in her own tears.

It felt good to hold her. It felt good that she responded to him. How long had it been since Marsha gave any response to an embrace? He'd missed that, but didn't know it until now with this stranger clinging to him.

"I don't know how much more I can take," her voice was squeaky and high, fighting sobs. "My husband has Alzheimer's and it's been so bad for so long. Everything goes wrong."

"I know, oh God, I know very well, all too well really. But we'll get through this." Jack spoke softly as he patted her back, "My wife has that awful disease too. Are you ready to get back up to the table and see what's going on? By the way, I'm Jack. Jack Rutherford." He offered his handkerchief and she carefully wiped her face with it. She sighed.

"I'm Anna Schmidt, and yes, I guess I'm ready." Her voice was steadier now. Even with red-rimmed eyes, she looked good.

She looked fit, as though she worked out regularly. Jack laughed at his own thought—he knew that anyone taking care of an Alzheimer's person worked out several times a day. Marsha's small frame and increasing thinness made it pretty easy for Jack to assist her. Anna's husband, while obviously wasted, still must weigh a lot more than she did.

Jack rose awkwardly, bumping his head into the table top, then put out a hand to Anna to help her up. She came to his nose height, so that meant she was about 5' 6" or 7". So different from Marsha, who was only five feet tall. He had lost almost two inches of height from his tallest, and Marsha had lost about the same from her max of 5' 2".

Anna held Jack's hand firmly, finally

whispering, "Thank you, Jack."

She sat down at the table and held a napkin to her water glass, tilted it to wet a napkin, and worked to clean her husband's shirt and pants, which bore oatmeal, milk, and crumbs. She still had Jack's handkerchief and held it up toward him as if asking permission to use it in her cleaning. Jack nodded assent.

A young woman, perhaps a volunteer worker, came to their table. "I've called someone to clean the floor and I'll be glad to get replacement food for what is lost."

"Oh, thank you. That would be great," Anna said. "He had oatmeal, milk, and one slice of wheat toast. Oh, and a little container of jelly for the toast please. Any flavor."

Jack looked at Anna's eyes. They were the bluest blue he'd ever seen.

Indeed, those eyes were only a part of her good looks. She must have been a beauty when young, he thought. Actually, she still looked great even though a bit care-worn and tear-stained.

A prominent scar curved down from the scalp above her left eye and ran straight across her forehead to the hairline at her right temple. Maybe it continued into her hair at both ends. The scar couldn't be too old since the center looked reddish. An old scar would likely be a white line.

No one seemed to have paid any attention to their under-the-table drama, though Jack felt very conspicuous while down there. He expected a crowd might gather and ask questions. He knew he had no answers if that happened.

Looking at Anna as she introduced Karl, her husband, Jack judged her to be somewhat younger than he'd first thought. So here we have a foursome of seniors, half of us suffering from Alzheimer's disease, he thought. Well, half so far. One isn't interacting with the world at all and the other's being a troublemaker. One spouse is mighty troubled and I'm just an onlooker.

He and Marsha had gray hair, his quite a bit darker than hers. Karl's shone silvery white. Maybe Anna colored hers blond instead of letting it go white.

The replacement breakfast arrived and Karl attacked it. Anna let him mess around with it, but kept a grip on his tray. He fed himself much better than Marsha could. Anna kept wiping spots where the spoon missed his mouth.

"I can't think of any song words to fit the occasion," mused Anna.

"Song words?" Jack raised his eyebrows quizzically.

"I have what I call a jukebox that plays in the corners of my mind. That's from a song too, by the way. Anyway, I remember songs, or parts of songs; I might not know the whole song, but I usually know their names and some parts and pieces. Mostly old songs, but a lot of them."

Jack remained quiet for a while, then suggested, "How about the song 'Smile'? I don't know the whole song either, but it goes something like this: Smile. What's the use of crying? You find that life can be worthwhile, if you smile."

Anna rewarded Jack with a huge, beautiful smile, "Yes, I remember that one. I can almost hear Nat King Cole sing it. Thank you, Jack, that fits perfectly." Her voice now had a musical lilt.

Anna glanced at her watch. "We have to move on. Karl needs to stop at the lab, then he has an x-ray appointment. He didn't get much breakfast and he'd been fasting for the blood work early this morning, so I'd better take the toast and jelly along in case he wants more."

She wrapped the toast in two napkins and put it and the jelly in her purse.

"They're doing a lot of tests on him because he's participating in a research program here at The Clinic."

Jack asked, "Is Karl going for an MRI and other tests today too? And does he have neurological testing scheduled at a separate Alzheimer's unit later?"

Anna looked up in surprise. "I get it! Our spouses must be in the same program. This is great! I mean, I don't know anyone else going into this, and I feel I know you now. It's going to last all week. After the mess, I didn't think I could face it. I was ready to turn around and go back home. You've been very kind. Thank you."

"We're at the Travelers Inn, an easy walk to The Clinic building," said Jack, "but I hear it's a few miles to where we will be the rest of the week. Where are you staying?"

"We're at the HighWay Motel, quite close to where we'll be the rest of the week. It's quite a ways from here, as you just said. There are several motels near ours."

"Since Marsha and I are making the same stops today, we'll likely see each other again. I'll have to look at her schedule. There are so many appointments, I can only think of the last one and the next one. I don't even know the next one right now. But all are in this building or very close."

Anna reached to shake his hand in farewell, but Jack pulled her into a hug instead. "We are huggers where I come from," he smiled down at her. "You're a good hugger too." How good it felt to hold her again, much better without the tears.

Jack watched her walk away. She stood up straight behind Karl's chair, not bent over at all. He could almost hear Frank Sinatra singing 'You'd Be So Easy to Love'. This song business was contagious! The title words kept circling in his mind. Being with Anna would make waiting time pass quickly. He thought about what it would be like were he here alone with Marsha. It was good that they'd met the Schmidts.

2   Anna

Anna got Karl to his appointments on time. Not easy after that episode of losing it completely at breakfast. She'd felt at her wit's end during and after the drive to Rochester. Karl's worst behavior had gone on and on, making it a miserable trip. What should have been a six-hour drive at most, counting a couple of rest stops, had taken nine and a half hours!

They didn't get to their motel until after ten last night. Getting Karl settled took another hour and a half, then he'd had a wakeful night, getting up several times. He needed help in the unfamiliar motel room, so she'd gotten little sleep.

The scene in the cafeteria this morning was the last straw. Now she could feel her spirits gradually floating upward from that dark hell where she'd been.

Anna checked Karl in at the radiology desk at 9:15. Looking around the crowded waiting room for a place to sit, she saw Jack standing up, motioning for her to come to him, and pointing to a vacant seat and space enough for two wheelchairs next to him. She gladly joined Jack, hugged him lightly and thanked him for saving places for them.

Anna noted that Jack looked good, lean but with a little spread around the waist, thinning gray hair above an interesting face highlighted by a great smile showing perfectly aligned white teeth.

Anna said, "I must apologize for earlier this morn…"

"No apologies," interrupted Jack, standing and taking her hand, "I understand. The important thing is how are you feeling now?"

Anna answered slowly, "Better,

thank you. Maybe I got it out of my system. Getting here took a lot of effort.

"Being at The Clinic seems different or foreign, and we've been here several times over the years. We dealt with different health problems, like Karl's high blood pressure and my gall bladder surgery. I really had it this morning when Karl slathered his breakfast all over. Your understanding and help made all the difference."

Jack reached to touch Anna's arm, "You can relax for a while here. A staff member will take Karl and return him when they're finished. A woman took Marsha just before you came. So we'll be waiting a while. You've said you had a rough trip here. I guess you drove?"

"Yes. I do all the driving, of course—have for years. I'd looked forward to getting out and seeing different walls, different roads, different everything for a whole week."

"Did something happen to make it bad? Car trouble?"

"It's a long story. Are you sure you want to hear it?"

"Go ahead. We've plenty of time."

Anna recounted the whole trip to Jack; all of that wretched yesterday, thinking that might help ease the memory of it. She started with her early rising to finish preparing for the long drive from their home in upstate Minnesota to The Clinic.

She had packed Karl's wheelchair and two bags in the trunk of the old Buick the night before, so only their toothbrushes, a Thermos of coffee, some sandwiches and several snack foods were added in the morning. Getting Karl up, showered, dressed, and breakfasted took over two hours, but that wasn't unusual.

Anna saw next-door neighbor Thelma Jensen come out of her house and called to the pleasant 90-year-old. "Thelma, we're soon ready to go. I want you to keep a house key while we're gone." Anna walked over to meet her.

"Of course. What can I do for you while you are gone, Anna?" Thelma asked.

"Would you take in my mail this week? We should be back Sunday." She fished in her purse for the extra house key intended for Thelma and handed it to her.

"Have a safe trip. I hope they can do something for poor Karl." Thelma wagged her head sympathetically.

"I'm afraid it's too late to hope for any big improvement, Thelma. I wish they could keep it from getting worse. We're invited to take part in a week-long clinical research study of those going into the more severe stages of Alzheimer's. Maybe others could benefit from what they find out."

"I'm glad you see it that way, Anna. I think you do a great job with him, but it must be awfully hard. How many years has it been since he started these strange things? I remember the old Karl so well—hard to believe how different he is now."

A distant look came to Thelma's eyes as she continued slowly, "I remember when he left your house and came to mine and no one knew where he was, including me! That was so worrisome. Not just me. Everybody was worried about him. I didn't know until the next day that he'd fed himself from my refrigerator and gone to sleep in my spare bedroom upstairs. I was here the whole time! Half the town was out looking for him. It got to be after dark and..."

"Thanks, Thelma," interrupted Anna, "I'll see you again soon. We really have to get going now." Thelma loved to talk, so breaking away from her always presented a challenge.

Entering her house one last time, planning to walk Karl to the car, Anna realized it was almost noon. It made sense to eat something before heading out. She gave Karl soup and half of a ham sandwich. She nibbled at the other half, looking around and thinking how much the beautiful old Victorian house had shrunk.

When Karl couldn't climb stairs any more, they contracted all their activities onto the ground floor. Gradually, the space they used became smaller and smaller. It was like being crushed slowly in a garbage compactor truck. Now the rest of the house contained dust-laden furniture and lacy cobwebs fashioned by occasional intruders.

The spacious dining room that once hosted family and guests at a large, beautiful, mahogany dining table surrounded by chattering, laughter, and squeals of delight over well-prepared food now served as Karl's bedroom. A hospital-type bed with side rails helped Anna know when he was trying to get up at night.

That dining table now leaned against a wall in the garage, its amputated legs lying nearby. When was the last time the sound of laughter warmed that room? She couldn't remember.

A sofa from upstairs fit into the open end of the kitchen, providing a good place for Anna to sleep and still keep an eye on Karl in his bed.

She missed sleeping with Karl. They'd slept with no space between them, cuddling close. But that had become difficult as his disease set in.

He'd sometimes become agitated in his sleep, lashing out at whatever demons attacked while he slept. He would awaken and continue fighting against objects around the house. He didn't attack me then.

Anna endured confinement to the home and the immediate surroundings like a prisoner awaiting an indefinite death sentence.

They bought the house when the boys were young. The walk between the house and the hardware store Karl owned took five minutes. How long would it take to walk Karl there today? There was no connection to the store any more. In fact, they had few connections to anything or any one any more.

Feeling time pressure, Anna left the dishes on the table and got Karl up to walk him down the ramp and to the car. Mark Miller, a nice young man in the neighborhood, had built the ramp with a fine handrail as his Eagle Scout project. So many things needed changing to meet his needs.

As Karl took one unsteady step after another, Anna looked around at the remains of a yard once filled from early spring through fall with masses of blooming plants. Not this year—and not for many seasons before this. Anna used to spend hours each day making that yard beautiful. Now only some peonies, lilies, and a few unkempt rose bushes colored the grounds. The yard shouted "Neglect!" to any observer.

Settling Karl into the passenger seat took time. She needed to fold him just right and carefully help him lower himself into the seat. Karl's body permanently folded now, with his head leaning sharply forward and down all the time. It seemed to try to form an "S". The next task involved lifting each of his legs and turning them to get his body facing forward inside the car. Finally she closed the car doors.

Anna started the 300-mile drive anticipating the pleasure of being somewhere else. Thelma's long visit with her incessant talking this morning had put their trip behind schedule. Few people took time to visit with Anna, so she should be appreciative.

Over the years of Karl's illness, Anna became her own best friend. She talked to Karl a lot, but he didn't often respond in a way that showed he understood her. He talked little now; just single words or short sentences, often unintelligible.

Karl sang though and seemed to remember song words amazingly well. Even though he had sung since childhood and knew hundreds of songs, she thought it curious that he remembered songs and almost nothing else. Anna thought he still sang almost as well as when he had been at his all-time best, and that was at the level of a professional.

Anna's thoughts abruptly changed course as the seat belt buzzer raised its alarm. How had Karl unbuckled his belt? Another new behavior. New and not good. Why did he do these things? Anna stopped the car alongside the quiet road to rebuckle Karl.

"Please Karl, don't even *touch* that buckle again."

Within a minute after getting underway, the buzzer sounded a second time. Again Anna stopped. The third time it happened, Anna shouted, "I've asked you to leave that seat belt alone. Now STOP IT!"

Karl smiled at her. Anna thought his deep brown eyes expressed impishness. The thick coal-black eyebrows above them contrasted sharply with his silver-white, wavy hair. He seemed to be enjoying this unbuckling game. Did he know when he annoyed her? Did he mean to do it?

Peace and quiet reigned for about half an hour. Karl dropped off to sleep, but soon awakened again. He turned the radio on and the volume up. Not just loud, but blaring music with a fast hard beat and gruff, offensive words—nothing Anna wanted to hear.

"Please, Karl, not so loud." Anna reduced the volume and scanned the radio for something pleasant. Karl, the gifted vocalist, usually enjoyed listening to music in the car. A Mozart concerto calmed Anna for less than a minute when Karl again changed the station.

Another hip-hop number, this time with few understandable words, jarred her nerves. Had Karl remembered the station number and deliberately turned to it? No, that couldn't be possible for a man who couldn't operate the toaster or remember his own name, let alone any numbers. She found the Mozart again.

"Anna, meine musik! Bitte lass mir." Karl pulled at her arm.

Karl used German more and more often. Some of it she could understand—not the exact words, but his meaning. "Meine musik" translated easily to *my music*, but the other words meant nothing to her. Karl learned English after he began grade school, but he had spoken almost no German since childhood. Why now?

Anna tried persuasion, coercion, humor, and threats. Karl kept fiddling with the radio, stopping at the hip-hop station whenever his fingers found it. He had *never* liked that type of music.

She stopped at a rest area and extricated Karl so that she could walk with him for a while and change his pad. He needed exercise and it might help take his mind off the radio and that awful music.

Finally underway again after about 20 minutes of a good walk followed by a snack of Wasa bread and an apple, Anna hoped for peace and quiet. Almost immediately, Karl fiddled with the radio, hunting for "Meine Musik, bitte."

In college, Karl majored in business and music. He'd been a soloist in the college choir, which presented performances on campus, on U.S. tour, and even in Europe. Before Alzheimer's gripped him, he was in demand as soloist for weddings, funerals, and public events in a wide area around Bemidji. His fame exceeded that of Pavarotti, at least in parts of Minnesota. His huge repertoire included classics, Broadway musicals, oldies and newies, but never hip-hop.

How much did Karl regret not trying for the life of a professional singer? He must have, at least a little, but he'd never complained. The family hardware store needed him and it took priority over any other ambitions.

"I wonder if there is somewhere under the radio I could disconnect a wire or do something to shut it up for the next few hours," Anna muttered.

"Karl, I know what you want. Let's just turn it off for a while." The tension grew as the miles slowly ticked off on the odometer. Anna tried to distract herself by redoing words to the song, "But Not for Me".

The things I'd like
to hear and see
Are not for me.
My song goes on,
I'm not lucky.

"Well, Anna," she said to herself,

"You've got to stop it now. You're feeling sorry for yourself and that doesn't help anyone." Funny how often she talked to herself, and out loud too. No one listened. No one responded.

She caught a glimpse of Karl reaching down to release his seat belt buckle yet again and grabbed for his hand. The car swerved slightly, but was in control immediately.

Blue lights flashed in the rear-view mirror. She wondered what emergency brought a police car to this quiet stretch of road. The car didn't pass, so Anna braked and steered to a stop on the right shoulder to wait for it to go on. It didn't. Instead it pulled up close to her rear bumper. Now she could see it was a state patrol car.

A very young uniformed officer emerged and walked up to Anna's window. Sighing heavily, Anna rolled it down.

He asked for her driver's license and car registration. She fumbled the license out of her billfold and wrestled past Karl to reach into the glove compartment for the registration, protesting, "I haven't done anything wrong."

"You were weaving all over the road, ma'am. Very unsafe driving."

Taking a deep breath and trying to calm herself, Anna addressed the young man, "Officer, I swerved very slightly one time, but I was NOT weaving all over the road. You see, my husband has Alzheimer's and his behavior this morning is unusually disruptive. I'm just trying to safely get us to appointments at The Clinic."

"Safety-minded? Well then, why is your passenger sitting there without a seat belt?"

Startled, Anna looked to her right. Sure enough, Karl's seat belt draped his right shoulder, with the buckle shining on his chest. Karl beamed a grin at Anna. With the car's engine off, no buzzer had announced his offense.

"See that, officer? That's what he's been doing—unbuckling his seat belt every few minutes. I've stopped to fasten it three times since we left Bemidji. You must have seen that I drove slowly."

"I'll have to give you a ticket. It is not for speeding. You really need to fix your problem before you get a second ticket today." He started writing in a small book.

"Officer, you don't understand. I am simply trying to take my sick husband to a medical appointment. We are in a special study and will be there for a full week. He has Alzheimer's, as I said, so there are many difficulties and complications in the simplest tasks. It has been difficult to get him ready, to get him into the car, to…"

   "Lady," the young man interrupted, "I don't need to hear your story. You were driving unsafely and with an unbelted passenger. You now have a ticket for those offenses." He handed her the piece of paper on which he had been writing, turned, and strode back to his patrol car.

   Anna fumed, "Rude! Impertinent! Such an arrogant young man—no consideration at all." Anna wrapped her arms over the steering wheel and rested her head on them for a minute. "What kind of parents brought him up? There isn't a trace of mercy in that young law enforcer."

   Gradually Anna calmed down and got Karl buckled again. Looking at her watch, she knew she must resume the journey, but no sooner was the car underway again when Karl performed another successful unbuckling.

"That patrolman was right about one thing. I do need to fix the problem. Maybe taping the belt in place would work, but there's no tape. I'll try to find some in one of the towns we pass through," Anna planned aloud.

She wondered what Karl would do about such a problem when he was well. He had excelled at solving problems of all kinds. How she missed that Karl!

Anna sang a couple of lines:

There's nothing left for me
of days that used to be.
There's just a memory
among my souvenirs.

"What is the name of that song?" Anna shook her head, "Those words tell what's happened to Karl—no memory is left for him. Memory is so important and his has gone through a cross-cut shredder. He has no past. Things don't make sense to me any more, let alone to Karl."

As driving continued and Karl was quiet, Anna made up new words to one of her old favorites and sang again, this time with more vigor:

This is NOT a sentimental journey
They're gonna study his disease.
It won't be a sentimental journey
It's about loss of memory.

At Nisswa, a little town along highway 371, Anna pulled up to a small gas station to ask for duct tape. The attendant had none for sale, but gladly gave her a foot-long piece cut from a roll he kept in the back room. Gratefully, Anna taped the whole length of tape around Karl's fastened seat belt buckle and resumed the journey.

"OK, Karl, it's going to be a problem to get that tape off again and there will be sticky stuff left behind, but maybe we can have peace and quiet for the rest of our drive." Anna welcomed the engine noise, unaccompanied by any other sounds.

Karl's head fell to his chest as he dozed off soon after they started moving again.

"So that's the long play-by-play of our trip to The Clinic yesterday. I feel better after telling it, even though I probably bored you with the story."

Jack held both her hands, "You had a terrible day and then you said the night continued the stress. I think you've done very well, Anna. I'm sure we've both dealt with disappointment, sorrow and anger lots of times."

"What I didn't include in my story is the fact that when the patrolman left, after adding to the wretchedness of the day Karl had twisted into misery, I sat at the steering wheel, hit it with my fists, and swore 'Damn Alzheimer's! Damn that disease!'"

3   Jack

When Marsha finished in radiology, Jack took her to the MRI appointment. He carefully chose a place to sit in the waiting room so there would be spaces for Anna and Karl should they come here. He hoped they would. Time talking together made him feel better and he hoped that might be true for Anna too. In fact, he was sure it was. A caveat—this might be true just for today.

The breakfast problems added to the miserable car trip hit her hard. The moral? Make the most of today.

He picked up a *Smithsonian* magazine and tried to interest Marsha in some pictures. She just twisted her wedding and engagement rings and ignored everything else. He then leafed through another magazine, looking up every other page to see if the Schmidts might be coming. It was a short wait.

"You got here first," Anna parked Karl next to Marsha's chair.

Jack smiled with pleasure at seeing Anna. "Hello. I missed you. We've been apart for almost 20 minutes!" Jack felt he couldn't get enough of being with Anna. Some song words flitted through his head: Can't take my eyes off of you. That fit. Such blue eyes she has!

Her green outfit was set off by green dangling earrings and a short white scarf worn loosely around her neck, but secured with a brooch of the same green stones as in the earrings. He hadn't noticed that before.

How long had it been since Marsha had dressed attractively? Jack dressed her in sweats because they were easy to get on and off, important because he had to change her frequently.

He had to respect Anna's ability to take care of her own appearance while taking care of Karl. He unconsciously tucked in his shirttail. Maybe he should have worn a tie. No, ties were mighty uncommon among patients or visitors. The doctors used them but surprisingly, eschewed the traditional white coats.

Karl shouted, "Ach mein Gott! What's going on? What are we waiting for?" He twisted and turned to look around in all directions. Anna stroked his arm and gave him a magazine that he opened and closed over and over again, but didn't seem to look at. Then he tossed the magazine to the floor and reached toward Marsha's hand. He laid his big hand over her small one gently and was quiet.

Jack didn't trust Karl. Too erratic. Too temperamental. Better keep an eye on him in case he might hurt Marsha. Without warning, he flared up, but then gentled down.

"I feel off balance." Anna said.

"Dizzy?" Jack frowned with concern.

"No, I mean the way things change so fast with Karl. Just when I feel I've adjusted to one thing, something else happens. Something else to worry about, work around, accommodate."

"Yes, all the time, that's how it is. I've read a lot about Alzheimer's, but I never feel prepared for the things that happen. I want signs of improvement, but when I think I see some, it turns out to be more in my imagination than in Marsha's body. I'm always disappointed, even though I know the direction is downhill all the way." A silence fell like a gloom cloud over them.

Anna broke the silence, "Did you get a brochure about this MRI they're having, Jack?"

"Yes, the desk clerk gave me a brochure that explains how it's done. I guess you got one too. She said it would be different for those in our study group though."

"Why is theirs different from what it says here?" Anna wrinkled her brow.

"Well, because the machine encloses the patient and makes a lot of noise. It bothers a lot of people to have it done. For a claustrophobe, it would be tough.

"Our group is having head MRIs, so I guess they will be totally in the machine, and even though they use earplugs, there is noise and a strong vibration. It's loud and thumpy. So the operators will take more time before starting to acquaint them with the machine and put them in and out of the machine a couple of times. They will hear a recording of how it will sound too, just to see how they react to it."

"I wonder what they'll do if Karl gets upset. He's likely to do that, you know."

"They might give him a short-acting tranquilizer. They won't if it isn't needed. I don't think Marsha will be bothered. She goes along with whatever is going on pretty well, as you've seen. The bottom line is that this is going to take quite a lot longer than anything we've had so far."

"They seem to know what they're dealing with in Alzheimer's people, but I can see others are freaked out by it too." Anna shivered, "I'm glad I won't be in there when they do this test."

A young woman came to take Marsha to her MRI. When she started to wheel Marsha away, Karl shouted, "Back! Zurück!" looking at Marsha. They all ignored him and the staff member whisked Marsha away without another word from anyone.

Anna's eyes followed them. "I wonder what that 'Back' shout was about. So much I don't understand. When he first became ill, I didn't want to believe Karl was having serious trouble. All these behaviors made no sense for who he was and what he was for all his adult life before...before this. He lost his keys once. We never did find them. He'd forget names, get confused. He would get so angry and frustrated. Sometimes he'd lash out. He broke a chair once. Threw it against the wall."

"That must have been frightening."

"Yes, it frightened me. He hurt me once. That's another long story. I'll tell it to you if you'd like and if we have lots of time. Actually, Karl's calmed down a lot from the human fury he embodied at its peak.

"Our two sons took turns coming to help with him for a few months when things were getting difficult. Good thing.

I couldn't handle him physically, and it was pretty easy for the boys. Back then they related to their father as he had been when they went off to college. Now they come rarely and seem afraid."

"Of him?"

"I don't think it's fear of him. They're afraid they're at risk for Alzheimer's too. They say there's a hereditary factor. It scares me too—for them, and for my grandchildren. If our sons are not with Karl, they won't think about it so much. And they like it that way.

They think I should have put their father in a nursing home long ago. Maybe that will happen, but I want to postpone it as long as I can."

They were interrupted again as a young man came for Karl. He went quietly.

Jack frowned, "I don't think I could

ever put Marsha in a...facility." He couldn't make himself say *nursing home*. The words sounded obscene.

"I keep thinking about how Marsha headed the senior prom committee in high school. Even then she could organize anything. She relished every detail of the event. Until this disease hit, she could've told you what every girl wore, and who she came with, the songs played, who danced with whom, all of it, and in great detail."

"You must have had a wonderful time."

"Oh, she went with somebody else! I've been a bit jealous of that guy all these years. Isn't that crazy? She kept her corsage pressed in her dictionary, so every time she looked up a word, she nurtured those memories."

Jack became quiet for a moment, then said, "Eventually the corsage became dry and brittle, and it crumbled. Marsha then put it in a plastic bag, but kept it in the dictionary even though more pressing couldn't make it any better."

Jack twirled his wedding ring. "Now I think of her…that way. A crumbled flower." He took his handkerchief from his pocket to blow his nose so it wouldn't look like he was about to cry.

"After she became ill, I sometimes put the corsage out for her, but she never once gave a sign of recognition. It lost its meaning to her."

Anna reached for his hand. "My Karl was always organized too, ran the family hardware store for almost 40 years. He prided himself on his records. Felt he could handle any business problem. That's what he said. Then he began to lose track of money. He'd pay bills two or three times or not at all. He overdrew his bank accounts several times. I think some people took advantage of him.

"If I hadn't hired a manager, we might have lost everything. Karl was furious with me for that. By the time I sold the business, however, he didn't even know what I was doing. It went from bad to worse that fast.

"I had hoped one of the boys would come home and take over the business. That hardware store belonged to Karl's grandfather first, then his father.

"It would have been great to keep it in the family, but both sons have careers and they live about as far away as possible to still be in the same nation. Erik is in North Carolina and Otto in Oregon. Both are established in fields they prefer to a hardware store in their old home town.

"Do you know that Karl kept walking to the store most mornings after his mind stopped functioning? Every morning for almost two years? Two years! It wasn't good for the business to have him hang around with his strange behaviors. A few tried to be nice to him downtown, remembering the good Karl, but..."

4 Anna

Jack hesitantly asked, "Since we'll have some time to wait now, this might be a good time for you to tell me the long story about when Karl hurt you. Caretaking can be dangerous. My situation is so different from yours in this respect. I don't mean to pry. So if you're not comfortable talking about..."

"You know, Jack, it feels good to talk about the way things have gone. It's a relief to say it to someone who understands. That's you. Yes, I'll tell you the story now. It's a skeleton that needs to get out of the closet for an airing."

"Good. I'm glad." Jack again reached for Anna's hand.

"It relates to the scar on my face," Anna sighed as she touched her forehead scar with her fingers. "You were right too, it isn't a very old one."

"It's a very distinct, curved line on your forehead. Like a surgical scar. What happened?"

"An accident. A terrible accident. Karl cut me with a butcher knife."

"Oh, my God, Anna," Jack exploded, "you can't be living with someone who could do that to you!"

"That's exactly what others told me after it happened. It got to be very messy. Not just the bloody mess at first, but the emotional, legal, and social aspects got very complicated." Anna's voice faded out with the last sentence. Jack squeezed her hand gently. They sat in silence for what seemed a long time.

"He didn't mean to hurt me. I am positive about that. Let me tell you how it happened." Anna resettled herself in her chair, letting go of Jack's hand.

"It was a few weeks before Christmas. We were in the kitchen and I was baking julekake; that's a Norwegian Christmas bread with candied fruit and nuts—a part of my Norwegian family heritage. Karl seemed in a festive mood. I remember thinking that perhaps the smell of the baking julekake mellowed him out."

"I've heard of julekake. Something like a German stollen, isn't it?"

"I think so. Anyway, Karl started singing, moving around the kitchen and swinging his arms."

"Just tell me the whole story, Anna. I promise not to interrupt again."

"Anna took a drink of water and continued, "Karl played the Pirate King in *The Pirates of Penzance*, a role he had played in college. That day he swashbuckled with the best of pirates. His voice sounded great. As good as

ever, and that's really great. Neighbors
a block away could have heard him, I
swear.

"The kitchen became his stage for
the Gilbert and Sullivan comic opera and
he starred. He became more and more
dramatic and vigorous as he went on. At
first I worried that he might run into
something and fall. I stopped what I
was doing to watch him and laugh. He
seemed to be having so much fun. I
clapped my hands as applause in time
to the music. Then he grabbed the
largest knife in our big wood knife
holder and started swinging it as he
danced around the kitchen.

"I didn't see it coming. I felt a blow
to my head and then there was blood
gushing everywhere. I thought the knife
cut my eye because all I could see or
feel was blood. Blood poured down my
face, my clothes, the floor, everything.
That day I saw red! And only red.

"Karl stopped still at the sight of the blood. He just stood there, staring at me. I think he was scared, but I don't think he knew he caused the wound. I felt myself getting dizzy, so I sat near the phone and dialed 911. Because of the blood on my face I couldn't see the numbers on the phone and had to try three times to get those three numbers right.

"I held a kitchen towel to my face, but I couldn't cover all the cut area and it gushed like a fountain. I guess I fainted, because the next thing I knew the paramedics were loading me into an ambulance. One said something about 'so much blood'. I thought of a song of course–the line from 'Mack the Knife' about a body oozing life. That body was mine!

"The medic held something against my head as we drove. I must have been out for a while. Next I found myself lying on a high table at our hospital with several people in masks around me. I don't remember leaving the ambulance.

"I heard Dr. McClintock, the surgeon, say that we should have a plastic surgeon, but that he would do the next best thing. He used small needles and the thinnest thread to put lots of stitches close together. He did a good job of it, as you and as everyone else can see.

"I was anxious about Karl. They hadn't brought him along. He couldn't be alone. I said they had to get him. A nurse patted my arm and said they would see to it that someone was with him.

"Thelma, my next-door neighbor, came over to stay with Karl, along with a policeman. I think the ambulance people filed a police report, thinking they had rescued the victim of a violent crime.

"It was violent, and that kind of violence constitutes a crime, so I guess it made sense to them to report it. Maybe none of the crew knew anything about Karl and his disease, but Bemidji isn't so big that people don't know things like that. The crime report caused big problems.

"The police did not want me to be anywhere near Karl. Karl doesn't do well with others or in other places, so I had to fight to keep them from carting him off to jail first thing. The doctor thought I should spend the night at the hospital because I had lost a lot of blood. I refused. Karl needed me."

"What a predicament to be in." Jack reached to hold Anna's hand again.

"It was bad." Anna shuddered. "It took a long time and a call to our family lawyer, but eventually I convinced them that we would be all right. A policeman insisted that I get a special lockable case for the knives and anything else dangerous."

"Ha," Jack interjected, "Any home harbors a lot of dangerous things. What isn't dangerous around a home, especially in the kitchen?"

"I had the same reaction. Maybe they wanted to fit the whole kitchen into a case and demand that I keep it locked. I bowed to their command and bought a gun case. We've never had any guns, but it satisfied them that I had protected myself with it. Truth is that case has never held a thing."

Jack shook his head, "What a terrible experience for you and for Karl too."

"It was just that one time–like so many other incidents. They come out of nowhere, happen, and go into hiding. You never stop thinking it could happen again, so you worry a lot. I worry more about what's coming next than what just happened."

"I know what you mean, Anna. Looking way back to what I'd call normalcy seems so far away that I wonder if it was real. Maybe I'd want to go back to whatever there was before Alzheimer's, even if it was terrible.

"Our life together, Marsha's and mine, was good. I'm sure of that. We loved each other, shared a lot of interests, and enjoyed being together. Now it's tough, and I don't like to think about the future because I know things will get worse. But please go on with your story, I know there's more."

"After the police, a social worker wanted me to put Karl in a nursing home immediately for my own safety. She set about that goal with determination. Sometimes she cajoled, sometimes she threatened, but total separation of the two of us had to happen.

"I hated her visits. I believe she wanted to see evidence of abuse with her own eyes. She would come at different times of the day and evening, telling me she just wanted to say hello. I felt her eyes examining both of us, maybe looking for blood. She didn't sit and visit; she walked around our living area during the whole time.

"They took out my stitches after about a week and the scabs all dropped off after another couple of weeks. I don't know how I endured those days. It gave the town something to talk about, you can be sure. That's what energizes small town citizens–something new to talk about, especially something violent. Maybe because violence doesn't happen much. Maybe they envy the R-rated movie plots."

"I've heard about small towns and their unique way of knowing everything about everyone and talking about it forever. At least that's what the Prairie Home Companion attests to." Jack smiled.

"It's all true—and more. This event motivated me to come here to talk with Alzheimer's experts. I need to better understand Karl's disease in order to plan our future. They must know better than I do what will happen."

"That's the core of why I brought Marsha too. What's going to happen to them? When might it happen? What's going to happen to us?"

5   Jack

"Hi you two, how's zit goin'?" A short man wearing a backwards baseball cap, a loud print shirt, blue jeans, and cowboys boots stopped directly in front of them.

"Excuse me?" Jack said.

"My name's Clarence. Moved here from Ohio not long ago. Great place to retire. Best health care in the world right here and ya know what they say about older folks—the only music they like is organ recitals." The man laughed uproariously.

"I have to ask ya, did you find that contact lens ya lost under a cafeteria table this morning?" He winked at Jack. "Or was there a little hanky-panky goin' on down there?" Clarence leered at Anna.

"I beg your pardon!" Jack erupted.

"I like the live music down in the big entry area, but ya can't hear it from up here. Need to go down to the bottom level where that big piano sits. Ya ought to spend some time there. Great music. All for free. Ya'd love it. And today my favorite pianist, Jane Belau, is playing— probably for a couple of hours mid-day. Ya gotta take that in.

"I'd like to help ya enjoy The Clinic and the town. I can suggest great places to eat, things to see, stuff like that."

He talked so fast—you'd think he was selling The Clinic itself. "Where ya gonna be next?" the little man persisted.

"Actually," said Anna, "we spend today around here, then we're going to another area for the rest of the week. I don't think we'll be going out much or sightseeing. I think we'll be kept pretty busy."

"Where you guys staying?" Clarence seemed determined to learn everything about them. Jack was gritting his teeth. He watched Anna smiling at Clarence and wondered how on earth she could do that.

"We're staying at the HighWay Motel near where we'll be for an Alzheimer's study...."

"Yeah, I know the place. Good friend works the desk there. Ya stayin' there too, Buddy?" Clarence faced Jack.

"No. I'll try to get a room closer…"

"Just relax, fella. I'll do it for ya. I guess ya might like a handicap room. If I don't find you again, just call the HighWay this afternoon and ask if they have a room reserved for you. I'm really glad to help ya out."

Without saying another word, Clarence clumped down the hall in his high-heeled cowboy boots.

Anna and Jack stared at each other, then Anna bust out in giggles, "I'll bet Ohio was sorry to lose *him*!"

Jack would like to send him straight back to Ohio, or better, straight to hell—immediately or sooner. "That man butts in where he's not wanted or needed. Now he's going to take care of getting us a motel room. I'd rather do it myself than have his help. What a busybody." With a tight fist, Jack slapped a magazine against his knees.

"Enough about Clarence whoever-he-is from Ohio. Tell me where you come from." She said she guessed he came from a sunny climate because she'd noticed a tan line on his arm around his watch when he'd adjusted the band.

"Thousand Oaks, California. What about you?"

"Oh, I'm sure you've heard of Bemidji, Minnesota!"

Jack looked puzzled.

"Famous for its huge statues of Paul Bunyon and Babe, the blue ox. We lay claim to a few of those ten thousand Minnesota lakes too. Are there really a thousand oaks in Thousand Oaks?"

"Yep. Numbered and protected. I like it there. Very California. By that I mean it's free and easy in style. I worked for Glean, the company famous for being very green, very clean, very committed to environment, and for being a great place to work. I can tell you it's all true.

"The whole company, and I mean the bosses, the workers, even the customers take good aim for the best product while causing no harm. They want to use business to inspire and implement solutions to the environmental crisis. That's unique."

"Jack, you don't sound retired. You sound like a salesman for Glean. Karl loved his store. No doubt about that. But he never lit up the way you do when you talk about your work."

"I was an accountant for them. I'd say a majority of the people who work there are true outdoors people, in spirit, in lifestyle, in everything. I am too, but not so avid as most. I liked camping and fishing, and we skied some. Marsha and I loved dancing and socializing with people of all sorts of backgrounds."

"We Schmidts had a busy social life too. Ours had two circles, the store and our church. In Bemidji those circles overlapped."

"Do you know that at Glean there are no private offices?"

Anna looked puzzled. "How is that

possible?"

Jack went on, "It opens communication when you don't close doors. And even though it can be distracting sometimes, it does work.

"Like here at The Clinic. Have you noticed that the doctors don't wear white coats?"

"No." Anna's surprise was evident. "I've been here many times and never really noticed it, but you're right. Nametags have their doctor labels, but you can't tell who does what from the way they're dressed. Why do you suppose they are different from the rest of the medical world?"

"I heard it's an old tradition passed down from the early founders of The Clinic. They believed the white coat distanced them from the patients. They didn't want that, so no white coats to this day."

"From what I've read," Anna added, "The Clinic shows its principles in all possible ways such as their ban on smoking. You've seen the magazines around the waiting rooms. Well, they only subscribe to magazines that don't carry tobacco ads. I admire that."

Jack asked, "What do people in Minnesota do for recreation?"

"They are outdoors folk too, both summer and winter. All those lakes make fishing, boating, ice boating, and skating popular. Snowmobiling is big too, with special trails for them around the state. Our family of four went snowmobiling for a week once in the northern part of the state."

"You have a bigger range of winter sports available than we do in Thousand Oaks." Jack smiled.

"Our winters make for a lot longer season, too," laughed Anna. "We're often described as Minnesota nice. That means helpful, caring, considerate people. I used to believe that fit all of us. When Karl got worse, the caring people disappeared, even our sons. Alzheimer's scares people. Even when I take Karl for walks, people who used to come to the store, people I thought were friends, don't speak to us anymore. I feel like a leper."

Jack couldn't imagine anyone not wanting to talk to Anna, but sometimes he knew that leper feeling. "Marsha had lots of friends, fellow teachers she ran around with. You know, one good friend of hers named Clara Jean kept coming to visit after she got…sick. One! Only one. I haven't said this to anybody, but I got very upset about that. I could see why, but I don't like it. Clara Jean quit coming when Marsha closed up completely. For her, it must have been like visiting a pet rock. Most of the time, I can put on a happy face no matter how I feel."

Anna sang, "Spread sunshine all over the place, put on a happy face. Tell me how you happened to bring Marsha here for this research study? It's a long way from sunny California."

Jack laughed. "Yeah. 1500 miles. Actually it's because of Nancy Reagan."

"Nancy Reagan?!"

"Yes. Marsha had a friend who was a friend of Nancy Reagan. Nancy's stepfather was a physician and she, Marsha's friend, talked about The Clinic all the time, so what Marsha and I heard was third hand.

"I wish now I had brought her here as soon as we had a diagnosis of early Alzheimer's. She would have liked to come here, but at home she resisted going to doctors. So I guess I feel guilty about that. And then maybe we're here because I'm a little desperate for some hope. I figured if she could get help anywhere, it would be here. I know the reputation this place has, but what I've heard doesn't compare with being here. This place is awesome."

The attendant brought Marsha out and Jack rose to meet her. "How was it Sweetie? I hope it wasn't too scary." The attendant said she'd been very cooperative.

"The morning is gone! I can't believe how quickly the time skipped away." Anna checked her schedule. "Maybe we can meet for lunch in the cafeteria when Karl's done. Hope to see you there."

She gave Jack a little finger wave as he pushed Marsha away. "So long."

Jack hoped they'd connect at lunch, and he wasn't disappointed. He had already started feeding Marsha when Anna found them. A young woman with

skin like a china doll's set their trays
down, then hurried off to help another
wheelchair patient. Anna told Jack that
her small blue cap identified her as one
of the Mennonite volunteers at The
Clinic. Anna knew about them from prior
visits.

"You remember the young woman
who got Karl's replacement breakfast
this morning? She is one of that group
too."

Anna looked around and laughed,
"We must've been quite a sight this
morning on our knees under the table.
Now I can laugh about crying!"

Jack laughed too, "I thought about
being watched and even looked around
when we stood up. No one seemed to
be paying any attention, and that
surprised me. I did *not* see Clarence.
Where could he have been to see us?
That man!" Jack grimaced.

"Maybe it looked as though we were practicing some strange religious ritual," Jack speculated.

"If there'd been red Jell-O, I would have suspected it was a Lutheran ritual," smiled Anna.

"Garrison Keillor!" Jack said. "I told you I've listened to his radio program."

"By the way, did you know Mr. Keillor's been here for medical treatment too?"

Jack raised his arms in homage to The Clinic. "You treat presidents, kings, and Keillor plus a few million more ordinary folks. Do your medical magic for all of us."

"If you follow the Prairie Home Companion, you know all about Minnesotans," Anna said. "I enjoy the program too. Did you know the name of the program came from a cemetery just across the street from the Lutheran college Karl and I attended? When Keillor saw the name Prairie Home Cemetery, he decided to use Prairie Home in the name of his radio program."

"By the way, how did Karl react to the MRI? Did he freak out?"

"Surprise. The assistant said he slept through the whole thing! I can't believe it." Anna sighed and leaned forward, chin in hands. "Lyrics to fit this morning came to me: Just in time, I found you just in time. Then it says: I was lost, nowhere to go. That was me just hours ago. You saved me, Jack. How can I thank you?" She looked at him intently.

"I thank you, Anna. It would be a lonely, strange place for me if we hadn't met."

As they talked, Jack felt a deep kinship with Anna. They had so much in common—concerns, experiences, doubts, hopes, ups and downs. Sharing their stories felt good. From breakfast through a long morning, and now through lunch, his world had changed. It seemed like an old, comfortable friendship. He felt *alive*. It was a wonderful feeling. He hadn't felt alive or wonderful in years.

They continued talking as they fed their spouses and themselves.

Karl wanted something, but Anna couldn't understand because he spoke German again. He showed his frustration through hand waving, body fidgets and frowning. Anna was able to calm him by stroking his arm and shoulder and speaking softly into his ear.

Lunch finished, they decided to walk a while during the 45 minutes free time before the next appointment on the schedule. Leaving the cafeteria, they heard lively piano music. They headed for it along with quite a few others. Something magnetic about live music pulls people to the source. Not just to hear, but to watch the artist produce it.

About a dozen people stood crowded around the woman pianist performing in the big, high, open area. Some were singing along with the music. Others watched from a short distance. Looking upward, more observers leaned over balcony rails above them for two levels, watching and listening.

The song 'Moments to Remember' at a nice pace made Jack's feet itch to dance. "Anna, would you dance with me?" She nodded assent and they moved their spouses to a side wall where they could see and be seen.

They started moving to the music in a little open area. How thrilling to hold Anna and move to the music. She danced smoothly. How good to hold her.

This wasn't just being alive; this was heaven! A pair of women added a vocal duet as the musician continued.

When other nights and other days
May find us gone our separate ways
We will have these moments to remember.

"Anna, we are enjoying moments we will remember. Making memories for our future. You dance beautifully." When the music stopped, Jack asked the pianist, whom Anna knew was Jane Belau, the person Clarence had mentioned, if she could play "Could I Have This Dance?" She knew it. In fact, she didn't have any written music at all. One of the men near the piano remarked that she knew them all and beyond that, could play all like an angel.

They moved into the waltz. "Anna, the next part of the song asks to have this dance for the rest of my life. That is what I would like—to dance with you forever. He tried some variations in steps and Anna followed him easily. People opened up a circle around them, watching. Jack knew he could keep going for the rest of his life dancing with Anna.

The song ended, and suddenly Anna startled. Karl's voice rang out with 'Oklahoma'. He leaned against the piano, but faced the onlookers, his audience. Ms Belau smoothly accompanied him. At the end, Jane said, "I remember you. We did that number together when you came here several years ago. It's a treat to hear you again. Let's do another number."

"I hate to stop Karl and I hate to stop dancing, but we have to go to appointments." Anna looked meaningfully at her wristwatch.

"Thank you, Jane. Wish we could stay here all day."

The four of them headed for the EKG area, which would be up a few levels. There Anna and Jack checked in at the desk, then stopped at a window wall overlooking where they had danced.

"Imagine that. Karl must have known that he had sung that song with Jane before. We've enjoyed her music on earlier visits to The Clinic."

"It's amazing. Dancing with you is amazing. Think of the memories we are making."

"Let's sit here while we wait, Jack. This is nice. Quiet. I guess you call these conversational groupings along this corridor." Anna settled herself in an armchair and Jack chose one close to hers, at an angle so they could talk easily.

"I like this little buzzer," Anna said, "It lets you know when they're ready for you and you can be anywhere in the area. Better here than sitting in the big waiting room. I like the view. Just look at the lovely glass pieces of art around us.

"It's interesting. Karl and I liked dancing too. We went dancing at home once a week for years, even when the children were young. It was our date night. After the children were gone, we'd go to polka festivals over two or three weekend days. A few times we used our vacation time to go to festivals farther away, some lasting a week or even more."

"Polka sounds pretty vigorous. Marsha and I did ballroom and liked the Latin dances. Never did the polka."

"Maybe that's a Midwestern thing. Lots of different European groups settled here, bringing their music with them. Poles, Czechs, Slovenians, Germans, each with polka music, but each with a somewhat different sound.

Different instruments, different pace, but you can dance the same steps to any of them. It's said to be the most aerobic of all dances. I'd like to learn Latin American dances, especially the tango."

"I'd like to teach you. Too bad we won't be here the rest of the week. I'm sure Ms Baleu knows some tangos."

"What had you and Marsha looked forward to doing when you both retired?"

"We both enjoyed our work worlds, but also looked forward to retirement. We planned so many things, things that weren't possible while working, including lots more dancing. We wanted to travel, do projects, and explore new activities to see what we both liked. She taught elementary school and loved working with the young children. I didn't understand it when she wanted to retire early."

"We didn't even plan retirement. Having our own hardware business, we thought we'd stay in harness until we dropped. Now of course that's changed with the Home Depots and Lowe's stores everywhere. We might have been forced into retirement."

"Your business timing may have been excellent, even though you were forced into it. I accepted that Marsha might want to stop working and do other things, but it took a while to see that she hadn't been able to handle things at work anymore. I don't think others were aware as much as she. She became super anxious about every lesson, whether planning it, giving it, or thinking about it afterward."

"Karl had anxiety too—over everything at the store. It seemed to run smoothly, so why was he so uptight? It didn't make sense to me. He's still anxious, I think. He fidgets and seems to want things and I don't always know what he wants, whether he's using English or German."

"Marsha lost sleep, lost weight. Finally, she felt she had to stop teaching for the sake of the children because she couldn't perform at her best and she couldn't accept giving them anything less. She got worse fast, and soon I saw that I couldn't wait for age 65 to retire, so I stopped at 62. She needed all my time and energy."

"Oh, don't I know that feeling! I've devoted myself to Karl, knowing that no one else would care for him as I could. I worry a lot about what happens to him if I die before he does."

Jack nodded, "I understand. That worry haunts me. We have no family who could help out. I've made arrangements, just in case, to be sure she's taken care of, but I think it would be hard. I hope that doesn't happen."

"We have family, but I know what they would do. Maybe later that would be OK. But for now...no, it wouldn't. In the earlier days, well, I'm not sure…" Anna gazed out the window.

"When I finally realized how sick Marsha was, I had to make huge adjustments in my attitudes as well as our lifestyle, and it was difficult. I resented it for a long time. How could she do this to me? Why just then, when we should have started enjoying free time?" He stayed quiet for a time and they both stared out the window.

"Jack, you are very up-front about your feelings. I don't think I've felt bitter toward Karl, but I hate the disease. I believe an evil monster came, took my husband away, and left this wretch with me."

"Wow, you said that well. That same evil monster came to our home too."

"We have so much in common, yet we met only this morning. It's like the song, 'Getting to Know You'. Anna sang, 'Getting to know you, getting to know all about you. Getting to like you, hoping that you'll like me.'"

"I like hearing you sing, Anna, and I like the words. Wasn't it a woman named Anna who sang that in the musical, too? Of course," he laughed, "the musical was *The King and I*. I remember now, that was from the book, *Anna and the King of Siam*.

"I feel I've known you for years. The part about liking you is true, Anna. I think we need each other."

"Do you know the song 'You Needed Me'? It says I cried and you wiped away the tears. That's what you did for me, Jack. That song is about mutual need. I wish I remembered more of the words."

"You know, Anna, songwriters do

society a great service – they say what we can't say easily. Words and music linger together in our memories longer than words alone. There they are, available to savor over and over.

"I don't think I appreciated that much before knowing you. Since you think in songs, I'm doing it too. Maybe songs will be our special language. Sometimes just listening to music serves as an anti-depressant for me."

"Most times I feel OK about things. I can handle it one day at a time. Times come when I feel down, though. It's as if the marrow has been drained from the skeleton of my existence," said Anna. "Karl's taken medication for depression. I've wondered if depression could be contagious. Do you think Marsha is depressed, or has been?"

"She may have been. Or Alzheimer's may be the cause of her introversion and quiet. Her doctors haven't said anything about depression, but I don't know. Since you and I started talking, I'm getting a new perspective on a lot of things. That is another thing I will ask about.

"Maybe I've been depressed and didn't know it. Now I feel alive, as if I'm back from the grave. I felt dead compared to what I feel today. Finding you makes such a difference," Jack blurted as he reached for her hand. He held it, wishing he could hug her again. But that would be too much too soon, he thought, so he just held her hand for a minute.

Jack wished again that he could have shaved. Marsha had always been so appreciative of a smooth face when he kissed her. His stubble made her face break out, beginning the first time he'd kissed her. So he'd made it a habit to shave really close and often for Marsha. He'd kept an electric razor at work to shave just before leaving. Then he could kiss her hello when he walked in the door at home.

Anna asked, "You and Marsha don't have children, Jack?"

"We had a daughter, Sarah, who died in infancy."

"I'm so sorry, Jack. That must have been terrible."

"It was. We hoped to have children for a long time, but gave up. Marsha became pregnant at 42 years old—quite a surprise, one she couldn't believe for months. She called herself Sarah and laughed as the biblical Sarah had. This happened at a time when most babies were born to mothers in their 20s and early 30s."

"I gave birth to our boys while in my 20s. Are you saying that Marsha liked the idea of the older Sarah so much that you named the baby Sarah?"

"Exactly. We'd gotten used to the sound of the name Sarah and the idea of laughter that went with it. We were giddy with happiness and laughed a lot. Marsha took a leave of absence from her teaching to stay home, care for, and breast-feed Sarah.

"I loved getting up to bring Sarah from her crib to Marsha at night or early in the morning. It was fascinating to watch the two of them together as Sarah suckled.

"Marsha always felt self-conscious about her small A-cup breasts from puberty to Sarah's birth. While feeding Sarah, her breasts enlarged a lot, and that really pleased her.

"We lost Sarah after only six months. She seemed to be a thriving, cheerful, smiling baby. Then one morning, I heard nothing from her. Usually she awakened at the same time every day. I went in to bring her to our bed. She was cold and still. Marsha called 911 and I tried CPR." Jack's voice broke. "No explanation, no reason for her death."

"How heartbreaking," Anna reached over to touch Jack.

"Marsha said her breasts grieved. They cried tears of milk for days. Tears from her eyes joined those milk tears. I suffered, but I know that grief gripped Marsha harder and longer.

"She often talked about those few months of being a C-cup person. The experience meant something to her. Once she had considered surgery to augment her breasts. I found her totally beautiful and cared nothing about her cup size. Her inner beauty shone through and I loved her very much.

"Marsha got to know her principal, a woman named Bobbie—her real first name. Bobbie's endowment in the breast area attracted lots of attention. Even the youngest kids in that elementary school called her Booby. She told Marsha how she envied women with small breasts."

Anna laughed, "We women are sensitive about breasts—when they appear, how big they become. It's size, size, size, and always the wrong size."

"Marsha memorized a poem by Roland Flint, a poet from Maryland, because it made her feel better. She called it an ode to small breasts, although Flint's title gave no hint of that emphasis. Flint wrote that he loves small-breasted women. One of his lines says small breasts never fade or fall."

"That's interesting. As I get older, I can appreciate those virtues of small breasts. I used to be a 36 B, but now I'm a 36 Long!"

Anna laughed as it took a moment for Jack to get the joke. "Maybe the sags are the payment we older women make for having had larger breasts when younger."

"I've never thought of the problems of the above-average-breasted woman, just knew how quickly Marsha would have traded with her."

"I just thought of something, Jack. Did the poet Flint come from this area, I mean the Midwest?"

"I don't know his origin. He taught at Georgetown University in DC—poet laureate for Maryland too, so I think of him as belonging there."

"Garrison Keillor, you know, the Prairie Home Companion man, and a poet from North Dakota, I think, did a benefit performance together after the terrible 1997 flood in Grand Forks. Karl and I attended.

"I'm pretty sure, now that I think about it, that that poet must be the same Flint. I heard some of his work during that program, including a memorable one about oysters and frustration. Nothing about women at all." Anna laughed and added, "*Consumer Reports* gives an annual Oyster Award for the packaging of a product that is hardest to open. I've wondered if that award was inspired by Flint's oyster poem."

"Well, if it isn't the cozy couple," came a comment from right behind them, floating into their conversation like a bad smell from a broken sewer. Clarence, clutching a newspaper, came from behind their chairs and walked around to face them. "How zit goin'?"

Oblivious to his disruption, Clarence ogled Anna's breasts and continued, "Jack, ya know, I'm surprised at ya. Men don't talk about cup sizes for hooters.

We talk about hands full or liken their boob size to food, not alphabet letters. Ya know, the babe has melons, or grapefruit or oranges, or for the gals who don't have it up there, it's fried eggs. Now, for Anna here, I'd say..."

"Where have you been, Clarence? You must have been close to hear our conversation," Jack interrupted, voice dripping disdain.

"Oh, I walk the floors here sometimes. Enjoy that. Found a seat right there behind you to read the paper." Clarence pointed to a chair whose back almost touched the back of Anna's chair. "Listening to ya guys made me think of a funny song about saggin' boobs. Do ya remember this kids' song?

Do your ears hang low; do they wobble to and fro?

Can ya tie 'em in a knot; can ya tie 'em in a bow?"

Clarence continued loudly if not melodically. "Well, I've heard it this way:

Do your boobs hang low;
do they wobble to and fro?
Can ya tie 'em in a knot;
can ya tie 'em in a bow?

He laughed as though he'd just heard the world's funniest joke.

Clarence had been there the whole time! Listening to every word. Why hadn't they seen him? Because Clarence's small stature could hide in that high-backed chair. Marsha might see eye-to-eye with him if she were standing, even in his high-heeled cowboy boots. When had he come in?

"You seem to like eavesdropping on conversations more than reading." Jack's voice iced over.

"Sure do! That's what makes this

place interesting. It's the people. Like you two and your wheelies. I've thought of being a regular volunteer here. They use lots of retired folks to help people out with information, directions and such. But I don't like to be tied to a regular schedule. Like my freedom, ya know.

"Now I've got good news for ya guys. You're gonna be neighbors at the HighWay. Got it arranged in a couple minutes with my friend, the desk clerk there. Did it over the phone. Didn't even have to drive up there. Since ya gonna be here a few days, I could help you with other stuff. Of course, that is, if you're not too tied up with each other…" he smirked. "I'd love to help ya out."

"You already did. Ms Belau's piano music pleased us, Clarence. You recommended it and we even danced to it," said Anna.

"Yeah, I saw ya makin' good use of

that music. Some pretty fancy moves too. I could tell y'all been practicin' for years."

"Anna, we'd better move in for our appointment," Jack rose and turned Marsha's wheelchair toward the main waiting area. Anna followed suit. Clarence received no farewell from either.

"How many more stops do you have here today?" Clarence fell in step with them. "Will you stay over the weekend?"

"As Anna told you, we'll be in another building for the rest of the week, so don't expect to see us again. Goodbye, Clarence." Jack moved faster, leaving the obtuse little man behind to ponder his next prey.

"What a character!" Anna panted, struggling to keep pace. "He's the bad penny that keeps showing up."

"Yeah, except he's not worth that much," Jack groused. As they moved along the wide corridors, Jack sputtered indignation. He looked behind frequently to be sure Clarence wasn't on their heels. "That is the most obnoxious busybody ever!"

"I think he's amusing, and probably lonely. He wants us as friends. You have to feel a little sorry for him, Jack. He got a room for you in our motel. That was helpful."

"Even the best intentions can't justify intruding on us."

6   Anna

The afternoon vanished quickly. The last visit of the day for both Marsha and Karl would be with internists who would assess their physical health through the results of all the tests and a complete physical exam.

Anna and Karl finished at the EKG station and arrived early for that last appointment. After Anna settled Karl in the computer area of the waiting room, she signed on to the only free computer of the six along the wall at an angle to the appointment desk. She looked up information on one of Karl's medications, then checked her email.

Jack's voice came over her shoulder, "Hello. I looked all around for your bright green blouse in this big waiting room, Anna. I'm glad to find you. I didn't think to check over here. Are you starting here or finishing here?" Jack pushed Marsha's chair next to Karl's.

"You know this is the first time you got to an appointment before me. I just figured out that our study group members all have the same schedule and they assigned us in alphabetical order. So Rutherford comes just before Schmidt.

"I believe you're right. That's what kept us together all day. Karl hasn't started here yet. We got here early. Just checking my email. Amazing how important that is. I keep in touch with family and friends more this way than any other."

"So do I, Anna. It's because I'm tied to home a lot, so most of mine concerns business things. Some people are more comfortable sending a short note than being with us in person, even if they live only a few blocks away. Being around Alzheimer's people is just too uncomfortable for some folks."

Anna agreed, "So hearing from the cowards is better than not hearing from them."

Jack knelt to better look at Marsha in her chair, "Marsha's very tired. I'm going to put her across those empty chairs so she can stretch out. That will give her better rest than nodding off sitting up." He lifted her as though she were a doll and carefully eased her down across four chairs.

"May I move Karl's wheelchair up close to these chairs? Then Marsha won't fall off should she move suddenly. I don't think she'll move at all, but we need to be cautious."

"Sure, Jack. Sounds like a good idea. With those brakes on, it won't be going anywhere."

Satisfied that Marsha's position was secure, he walked up to look over Anna's shoulder as she worked the computer keyboard. "Looks like you're out in the web."

"I was checking one of Karl's medications. I wonder if it might be contributing to his troublesome behavior or whether it would be worse without it. It's on my list of things to ask Dr. Osowski. I'm finished now. Would you like to use this computer?"

Jack was ready to settle into Anna's chair at the computer when they heard Karl.

"Meine Frau, meine liebe Frau, mein Schatz," crooned Karl. Anna and Jack turned to look at him. He had stretched far to his right to put his hand on the sleeping Marsha's shoulder. He kept singing the words softly, over and over.

"I can tell Karl is a singer, all right. You said meine Frau means 'my wife', didn't you, Anna?" Jack stroked his chin in thought.

"Yes, it does. I'm not sure about the other word, but this is strange." She felt crestfallen.

Jack stood up close to Anna, "It feels strange to me, too, to see someone referring to my wife as his wife. But it is your husband calling Marsha his wife and sounding as though he believes it and cares for her. She is sound asleep, so she doesn't know what's going on. I'm pretty sure she wouldn't get it if she were awake either. How are you doing, Anna? You look as though you're in shock."

"Until right now, I've always felt that Karl knew me, knew that I am his wife, even when he couldn't say or remember my name. A little story gives an example of this. Karl and our daughter-in-law Emily got along especially well, starting with the first time Erik brought her home to meet us. After he became so ill, she would spend time with him when they came to Bemidji. That was much appreciated, especially since Erik rather avoided Karl.

One day after taking Karl for a walk in the wheelchair, she hugged him and said, 'Karl, I love you.' Karl responded, 'I can't help you. I'm married.'

I liked that. That memory means a lot to me. It meant that he knew he had a wife and he was true to his wife. He didn't confuse Emily with me. Now to hear him call a perfect stranger his wife! I can't explain it, it just is. I don't know how to handle this."

Jack put an arm around Anna as he saw tears appear in her eyes, "I think I understand. It's as you said, it's the disease, not the person. So you can't put too much meaning into this. Tomorrow it might be someone else he calls his wife. It doesn't take away from the many years you have been and are his wife and caretaker. Anna, it's going to be all right."

"What can I say? I need a song. No words fit, but thank you for your words, Jack. What would I do without you?" She turned to him and let the tears fall on his shoulder. Jack held her, stroking her back, and said again the little phrases meant to be soothing, just as he had this morning under that cafeteria table. He had to smile thinking how much more comfortable to hold her standing up than on his knees.

After a few minutes, Anna raised her head to tell Jack she'd thought of some songs. "Maybe Stormy Weather, or Lover, Come Back to Me, or The Way We Were."

Jack laughed, "Anna, you and your songs. They all fit. Why do you suppose you think in song words?" They continued to stand with his arm around her.

"A good question. I've even asked myself that. For one thing, my mother loved popular music and sang it around the house as she did her work, or as she did anything, I guess. Karl used to practice singing songs a lot, so all my life I've heard thoughts sung to music.

"I'm a shy person, so the ready-made words are handy. Then I don't have to come up with my own words. It seems safer somehow. I've never made a special effort to memorize songs, in fact, I usually know only parts of songs, but the sense of the song seems to stay with me. I don't really have a good answer – or a song that will provide the answer." She had to laugh at that.

"I don't see you as shy, Anna."

"Can't imagine why. I've been crying on your shoulder twice today now and we've talked for hours, as though we're old friends enjoying a reunion. No, I don't feel shy with you, Jack."

"I'm so glad my shoulder's useful. We are old friends." Jack looked at his watch, "Our friendship's over seven hours old."

"I am grateful to you, Jack. You know that. Without you, I might have taken Karl straight out of the cafeteria this morning and driven home to Bemidji. You've been so kind and considerate to me. I needed you.

"I rarely descend into despair, but right now I'm having trouble," she confessed in a frail, choked voice as she accepted Jack's handkerchief for the second time today and cleared away the tear streams.

"Anna, I have strong, positive feelings for you. They're unexpected, but real. I question the realness of the scene before us. That pair has mainly sat around all day, not interacting. We have interacted for many hours. There must be a difference."

Anna continued to watch Karl and Marsha. Karl's crooning continued, but barely above a whisper. He, too, must be tired. "The most important event of the day is that we've found each other, Anna." Jack hugged her.

"And our spouses followed in our footsteps, or we in theirs, I wonder...think about it. They've been next to each other, at the same level, in their wheelchairs. Maybe that accounts for it. People in wheelchairs are apart from others by the difference in levels."

Anna's pager buzzed, so she gathered their things and moved Karl up to the nurse who was waiting to usher them in to see Dr. Osowski. Jack moved over to protect Marsha at her resting place.

"Anna, this blows my alphabetical order theory. You're first this time." He blew her a kiss as she left with Karl.

This was the one appointment where Anna needed to be with Karl and the doctor. The nurse went through the routine of collecting height and weight, blood pressure and heart rate information, then she helped Karl prepare for his physical exam by changing him into a hospital-type gown in a small dressing room within the examining room.

Anna waited on a sofa-like seat, thinking how nice it was to have someone else dealing with Karl's needs. She extracted a pen and a small notebook from her purse, turning to the page of questions she wanted to ask.

As Dr. Osowski quietly poked and probed and tapped and touched all over Karl's body, Anna was thinking about Jack. This friendship seemed so comfortable, as though it had developed over decades. Their situations were so similar, as though one household mirrored the other.

She had to remind herself again and again that all this had happened since breakfast early this morning. She must not read too much into it. She had needed someone and Jack generously offered himself. That's all it was. One person helping another when both people have the same needs.

Anna knew she was reeling from physical contact with this man. He had held her, touched her, and it felt wonderful. It couldn't be this place. The Clinic was familiar territory to her, and it didn't seem to qualify as a romantic rendezvous spot. "What is happening to me? Why is this all I can think about?"

Dr. Osowski finished the physical, and then reviewed the results of all the tests performed on Karl, and on his blood and urine. There were no surprises; Karl's physical health showed no new problems. It pleased Anna that the doctor answered all her questions as though he had all the time in the world. He made it easy to discuss her concerns. That was one of the reasons they came to The Clinic—the excellent quality of care.

Finished, Anna thanked Dr. Osowski and looked forward to getting Karl back to their motel. She knew he was ready for supper, a shower, and bed. Tomorrow would be another new experience, at a new and different place. Tomorrow could wait. Fatigue enveloped her too.

She stopped to buy take-out meals for supper and drove to the HighWay Motel. In their room, she settled Karl into a comfortable chair at the small table that served as the dining table. They both ate hungrily from the several containers of food.

"Karl, I'll get us some de-caf coffee in the lobby. I'll be right back."

As she walked into the lobby, she saw Marsha in her wheelchair and Jack at the desk. "Jack, it's great that you are staying here."

"You told me about this place and how convenient it is to the study building. That sounded good and I have to give Clarence credit. There are no vacancies here this evening. I almost wish we'd see him again so I could thank him for getting us a room. Didn't even have to pay for tonight at the Travelers. They understood my situation and were very nice about it."

"I was about to get some coffee. Maybe you two would join us for a cup in room 116. They have de-caf, but we're tired enough that caffeine couldn't keep us awake," Anna laughed. "We just finished eating a supper of things I bought at the market up the street."

"I'd like that. We ate near The Clinic, so just got here. We haven't been to our room yet," Jack glanced at a small envelope in his hand, "Ours is 114, so we must be very close."

Anna poured two more cups of coffee and found a little tray on which to carry the four full cups. "If you like condiments, choose them now."

Walking down the corridor, Jack kept looking at Anna. "Here we are, 114. Let me get your door, Anna. Your hands are full." He took Anna's key card from the tray and opened the door to 116.

"Karl, we have guests for coffee," she called into the room.

Jack said, "Give me a minute to stow these few things." He nodded to two bags hanging off the back of Marsha's wheelchair. Opening the door to 114, he put the bags on the bed. Trying the other door in the room, he found he could open it, but that just showed him another door inches away. That one must be opened from the 116 side. He knocked on the second door. Soon Anna fumbled with the lock on the other side, and they were face to face.

"Hello. Our rooms connect! This is very convenient." Jack lifted Marsha from her chair. "OK Sweet Cakes, let's get those legs moving." Together they entered the Schmidts' room.

"This is the first time I've seen Marsha walk. She does well."

"Her balance isn't great, but she has the strength to walk short distances. How is Karl at walking?"

"Like Marsha, Karl can walk, but it's difficult. He's unsteady and sometimes overreacts if a step doesn't feel right to him. Also, he's pretty heavy, so I can help support him in walking, but I can't lift him should he fall."

Anna gave Jack two cups of coffee,

and Jack added some cold water to Marsha's, then Jack and Marsha sat on the bed. He held her coffee cup and passed it to her mouth frequently. Anna went through similar motions with Karl at a small table across from the bed. They talked about the HighWay Motel and what they expected might happen at the study center in the morning.

"One problem I have with Karl is bathing. He loves sitting in a tub filled full of water. It's great for him, but it's difficult to impossible for me to get him in and out, so we usually shower together. There I can help support him and avoid falls."

"Marsha likes showers. We have a walk-in at home that we use all the time. We shower together too, like we have off and on since the early days of our marriage, when it seemed so romantic. Now it works just as you said. I can support her and we both get clean in no time. I know Marsha enjoys the shower, because she will sometimes smile then."

"Our shower at home comes from a shower head over the tub. Karl usually signals that he wants to sit down in the tub, but I can't let him do that."

"I've thought a lot about showers. It's sensual. Water a little too hot or a little too cold is uncomfortable. Just the right temperature's wonderful. Just like our coffee." Jack drank the last drop of his. "I've heard that Alzheimer's people are afraid of showers. I think it's because of that little difference in temperature that gives discomfort. One person's preferred temperature may be a little different from the next person's, so when two people shower together, one thinks it's comfortable and the other person thinks it's terrible."

Anna pondered a moment, and then said, "You may have something. I can tell that Karl does not like a shower. It could be fear, as you said, or it could be that I don't have the temperature just right for him, even though I am comfortable. We don't have a history of showering together to draw on to tell which is right."

"Anna, I have an idea. Karl could bathe in the tub in our room next door. I could help him get in and out of the tub."

"A deal, Jack. And you and Marsha can use the walk-in shower in our room. This room's equipped for the handicapped. I guess yours isn't."

Preparations for bathing Karl went smoothly. He settled into the tub, asking, "Meine Frau? Mein schoener Schatz?" a few times. When Marsha came back into the room and he could see her from the bathroom, he said it again several times, but without the questioning tone.

"Karl believes Marsha is his wife, all right. Can you get used to that?"

Anna said, "I'm better with it now. Maybe being attracted to someone is so basic that it can happen even with severe brain impairment. Some might say falling in love *is* a brain impairment!"

Jack guffawed, "I guess you're right. Whether it's goofy teen-agers or senior citizens, falling in love seems to derail the brain."

"For over a year in the earlier stage, Karl would make inappropriate moves on women—*really* inappropriate—with women at the store, women visitors at home, women he would see when we were out."

"How did those women react?" asked Jack.

"A few—very few, thought it was

funny. Most were scared to death of him. He couldn't be ignored. He was far too obvious and persistent in his actions. Strange, too, since he'd never done anything like that.

"Those things that are so out of character are hardest to understand, aren't they?

"Karl took pride in being considerate and proper to everyone, especially women. He was involved in all sorts of civic and church activities, so everyone was surprised that he could change so drastically, and that included me."

"Did he act differently toward you, too?"

"Yes, he certainly did. He wanted to make love all the time. Sometimes he could and sometimes he couldn't, but he seemed obsessed with the idea."

Jack lifted Karl from the tub and

soon Anna had him dry, freshly diapered, and in pajamas. Jack helped Karl into the big bed, then he and Marsha showered. Soon Marsha was ready for bed. "It's been a long day for these guys. I'll bet they both sleep well tonight." Jack and Anna sat by the table in Anna's room.

"Look at Karl, Anna. He's tapping the space next to him in bed, still saying meine Frau and other words I don't understand."

"Karl hasn't shown interest in anyone since that sexy period about five years ago. That is, until now, with Marsha, and that may not be sexual. Isn't that puzzling?" Anna frowned and looked concerned.

"Jack, a postmistress I knew told me that her father lived in an Alzheimer's unit of a hospital and that one pair there was inseparable. Always together and always touching each other. The man was a Roman Catholic priest! So again, you know it's the disease."

"Marsha had always been careful of what she said. As a teacher of young children, she didn't want any misunderstandings or for people to think she couldn't control herself. So we had the same kind of nasty surprise when she started cursing a lot."

"I can't picture Marsha cursing. Could you think of a reason for it when she did?"

"No. No reason. Nothing happened that might have made her upset enough to curse. She'd just start spewing out long strings of words I would have sworn she had never heard, let alone spoken.

"I worried about it for a long time. As with all the other things that are surprises, you feel it means something awful is happening in their disease. And it is. But this, too, stopped eventually and she's never gone back to it during the years since."

"Did Marsha go through a heightened interest in making love too? I've heard it isn't uncommon with Alzheimer's."

"No, she never did. Before her illness, I know she enjoyed our sexual relations. When she became ill, she seemed to pull a shell around herself, as though trying to hide. That's why her drunken sailor language surprised me so. She's normally—if I can use the word 'normal' within her illness— withdrawn and quiet. Early in her disease, when I made love to her, she seemed disturbed. It made me feel I was taking unfair advantage of her, so I gave up."

"Oh, Jack, look at the time. We do manage to talk for hours. In the morning we need to be at the center by

8 o'clock. That means breakfast first. They serve a good breakfast in the lobby–cereal, bagels, toast, fruit, even waffles, and it's a lot faster than going out."

"Anna, would you like to walk to the center in the morning? The desk clerk told me it's a little over half a mile. That adds only about ten minutes if we walk briskly. It seems to make Marsha relax to be outside and I need the exercise. We've been sitting a lot. It would be especially nice if we could go together with our wheelies, as Clarence calls them."

Anna looked at her watch again. "Let's put in a wake-up call. I need the walk too, but I don't want to be late. I never know how much Karl will eat or how much trouble he might make. I'm still spooked by that scene at breakfast this morning. Without you, this could have been as miserable a day as our travel day yesterday. You have helped me so much. I can't thank you enough."

"I'm grateful to Karl for his scene this morning," Jack reached toward Anna and lightly hugged her, "Without his help, we wouldn't have met until tomorrow when our group convenes for the study. He opened a special friendship for us."

They stood up from the table in Anna's room, ready to say goodnight. The moment melted away abruptly when Marsha came staggering into the room. Jack started toward her, but then hesitated, waiting to see what she would do. He and Anna gripped hands. He whispered, "Wait." Marsha walked to the bed and, with some struggle, climbed in beside Karl. She pulled at the covers as she awkwardly scooted herself closer to him.

"Another surprise." Anna looked stricken. "We knew Karl thinks Marsha's his wife. They've held hands this afternoon, but I thought Marsha might just be tolerating him. I had no clue that she shared the attraction. Did you, Jack?"

"Not the slightest. Let's stay here a few minutes and see what happens next. Karl is asleep."

"I could get some more coffee or tea if you like," Anna offered.

"No, thanks. With Marsha's surprise move, I'm fully awake again. We could visit as we keep watch."

"I feel pretty shaken, just to see another woman in bed with my husband. It's puzzling and more and more disturbing."

Jack examined Anna's chagrined face. "Yes, it is hard to see your spouse expressing affection for someone other than you. It's been a long time since

Marsha showed anything but infrequent smiles for me. She's always so distant." Jack explored facets of this new development and how he and Anna felt as they sat and processed this development.

"We are equally astonished and pained," said Anna, "To them this is good. How can we just ignore it?"

"Look," Jack rose from his chair and pointed to the bed. The couple there was curled up spoon-fashion, Karl's arm around Marsha, and both were asleep. "See how contented they look."

"I remember watching our children sleep when they were little." Anna added, "They, too, looked so peaceful and content. Then the minute they awakened, their energy stirred the household—peace displaced by constant activity. I suppose these two will be back to where they were in a few hours."

"I wonder if their attraction to each other will change them." Jack shrugged. "We'll soon find out. Maybe we'd better try for some sleep ourselves now."

Anna looked at Jack quizzically, "And where are we going to sleep? Are we going to separate the peaceful, sleeping duo?"

"No, I really believe in letting sleeping spouses lie. I have a plan. I always carry an air mattress in our van at home. Marsha tires easily, so she can sleep in the back when we are driving for errands. I brought it along to use in our rental van, thinking we might need to drive places and do things here too. I will sleep on it in your room. You can have our whole bed next door all to yourself. OK?"

"Jack, you are a generous, thoughtful, and prepared person. I appreciate and accept your offer."

7 Jack

Jack shut off the alarm when rays of sunshine peeked between the window curtains. He'd slept pretty well and now lay on his floor bed, looking forward to finding out more about the research study and what the week would bring. He heard stirring from Anna's direction and said softly, "Anna, are you awake?"

"Yes, I am." He heard her yawn. Maybe his voice awakened her.

"Sleep well?"

"Yes, great quality if not quantity. Karl was worn out from the long day yesterday and slept better than usual. Therefore he didn't awaken and need me, so I slept well too."

"Where do you suggest we eat? In the motel breakfast room or here?"

"Let's plan to eat here in the room.

After that, I'll shave Karl and get him dressed." She picked a gray sweat suit out of a suitcase. "They suggest casual clothing at The Clinic. That's all he ever wears anyway."

"Sounds like a good plan." Jack shaved, got dressed, and set four chairs at the little table. Even though he made noise, and Anna's moving about and showering wasn't exactly quiet, neither Karl nor Marsha stirred. He and Anna walked down the hall to the breakfast room.

Clarence, of all people, greeted them. "Howdy, ya two, how zit goin"?" Did I do all right by ya?"

Quickly Anna turned her back to Clarence and whispered to Jack, "Now behave. You said you'd thank him, remember?"

"Good morning Clarence. Everything is fine, thank you."

"Just thought I'd check. I sometimes come here to have coffee with my friend, and breakfast too, if nobody's lookin' too close."

"Good to see you Clarence. Have a great breakfast and a great day," said Anna. "As you see, we're taking breakfast to the room for us and Karl and Marsha. Then we're off for the day."

"I noticed ya didn't have your wheelies with ya. Thought you might have a breakfast-for-two date. It's fun to watch the two of ya. Overripe teens, that's what ya are."

Jack almost choked on that. He started to talk, but Anna pulled at his sleeve. "We're in a bit of a hurry."

"Don't let me hold ya up. I got things goin' today too. We'll see ya again 'nother time when we can visit."

Never had Jack put together a

breakfast tray faster. He added some fruit to Anna's tray to help hurry her along.

In the hall Jack exploded, "That man! We're shackled to him. I can't stand to be in the same room with him! The same building, even the same planet! What a jerk! Busybody! I'm saying a lot of other names for him in my head so I don't offend you, Anna. But don't you agree?"

"It was a surprise. Things must have gotten boring for him over at The Clinic. On the other hand, he does seem to have a special interest in us."

"Yes, he's our personal stalker! I'm so mad I'd like to hit him!"

"Really Jack, think about it. We are here and together thanks to Clarence. By the way, you did right to thank him." Anna opened the door to their room. "They said the Oyam Center, where we'll be from now on, practices tight security, so he's not likely to show up over there. I suppose they have to watch for impaired seniors escaping by accident more than check people who come in. It'll be OK, Jack."

They laid out the breakfast, roused their spouses and began the bathroom, eating and feeding routine. "Thank God we didn't bring them down to the lobby for breakfast there. We'd have to endure Clarence and certain indigestion."

Marsha didn't seem hungry, or maybe she was so used to her oatmeal breakfasts that she didn't want the cold cereal. Karl, on the other hand, seemed unusually hungry. Anna went back for a second serving of cereal and more juice for him. On return, she reported that Clarence had left the breakfast area.

"Good. I'm glad it's a nice day because I really look forward to our walk outdoors. It feels good to move and it always seems to be good for your Karl, even though he's not moving much. I think he behaves better after being walked outside. I'm glad Clarence is gone so I don't have to look over my shoulder every step of the way. Do you walk a lot at home? What about your Minnesota winter weather? I suppose that keeps you in." He switched topics, tired of steaming about Clarence and knowing Anna thought of Clarence with much more charity than he could ever muster.

"At home, I take him out a lot. Sometimes it's only in our own yard, but it's a lot easier to take him on the sidewalk or even the street. They clear the streets soon after a snowfall, so winter works too. Just the problem of getting a lot of outer clothing on and off. When we're out, some people stop and say a few words, especially if they are going in the opposite direction. Isn't that interesting? They can take the chance because they know it will be easy to move on when they've had enough."

"I haven't paid that close attention, but it makes sense. There is a park with nice walks near our home, so I walk Marsha there. I can leave the wheelchair along a path and walk with her on foot for part of the time. Then I get the wheelchair again when she's tired or doesn't want to walk. I'm ready to head out, are you?"

The four were out the motel door by 7:15. The weather reigned crisp and cool, but the sun promised warmth, given a little more time. Underway on foot, they could stride side by side on the wide walkway with sufficient space between the two wheelchairs. No one walked toward them. On the street, heavy early morning traffic drowned attempts at conversation. In half an hour they stopped at the entrance to the Oyam Center under a big sign reading "Welcome Alzheimer's Study Group."

"Let's take a few more breaths of this fresh air and go in." Anna breathed deeply a few times, then she and Jack pushed their partners up the rampway.

Jack thought, "Here I am. Here goes something. Here goes nothing. Wonder what will happen here."

Coffee, fruit, and muffins adorned a long table in the lobby. Could have had breakfast here. Their jackets and sweaters fit into a locker marked with their names. People moving to and from the table including several others in wheelchairs made it seem crowded.

At the lobby desk, they were given name tags and a schedule of the week's activities.

With cups of coffee in hand, they looked around. Jack saw confirmation that the study participants were chosen for their late stage of the disease. Marsha and Karl fit in, not just with each other, but with every other patient he could see.

Ten minutes before starting time. How many more people would be coming? As it turned out, they were the last. How could he forget that older people tend to be morning people and early to everything?

A rich collection of art enhanced the large lobby area. At least a dozen large paintings or drawings and three sculptures on stands begged their attention.

"Do you see the theme, Jack?" Anna asked after she had walked around and stood by each a short time.

"No, just a lot of interesting

artwork."

"I think each represents caregiving. Not all have a person as the care receiver. Notice the one of the child caring for an injured bird over there."

"How appropriate. You're good, Anna! It all comes together under caregiving, a unifying umbrella. I like it."

While still in the Oyam lobby, Dr. Krystyl Patel, principal investigator in their Alzheimer's research team, welcomed everyone and explained the schedule through Saturday. Smooth dark skin and graceful body and hand movements accented her youth as she spoke. She looked too young to be a doctor. Funny how many professionals seemed like children playing doctor. That attitude marked his own age, of course.

Talks and round-table discussions for caregivers supplemented the numerous neurological and psychological studies of the patients. He had said they'd be busy this week and the schedule assured him he was right.

Anna said she wanted to volunteer Karl for the sleep study. Like many Alzheimer's victims, his wake/sleep times didn't relate to day and night. That made sleep for their partners difficult, which made life difficult.

More than that, the sleep project would mean a full day, from noon one day to noon the next, when the patients would be with the project staff every minute. The facilities could only handle half of the twenty possibilities, so participation was optional. Jack knew an opportunity when he saw one, and this one was squarely in his sights.

Jack nudged Anna's arm, "Let's go over and ask to sign up right now before the formal programs begin. There might be many interested."

Together they approached a young woman holding a clipboard who handled the scheduling. Her nametag read "Inga Johansson, RN". She made him think of Freya, the most beautiful of the Viking goddesses. Her braided blond hair almost touched her waist in the back. Minnesota seemed to have a lot of blonds and their pro football team's name fit their territory.

Anna whispered to Jack, "How can we ask that they have the same day? We can't say we want time without them."

Anna and Jack signed the papers on the clipboard for their spouses. Jack told Inga, "If at all possible, please schedule these two together. They are very close."

Anna added hurriedly, "Karl believes that Marsha is his wife. He speaks to her in German sometimes. His parents were German immigrants, so he learned

German before English."

"Since you are the first to volunteer, I think that can be arranged, assuming there is no problem meeting all the criteria for participating. I'll give you a short questionnaire to complete. When that's reviewed, we'll notify you." The nurse handed them forms.

"Oh, Jack," Anna whispered, "I feel guilty. I wasn't considering what was in Karl and Marsha's best interests. My thoughts were only about what I wanted and I knew I couldn't ask for that. You amazed me when you gave an honest and logical reason for their enrollment together."

"I look forward to twenty-four hours of time we can use as we choose."

"If this works out, we can make use of some of that information Clarence gave us about what to see and do in Rochester. I wasn't paying close attention. Do you remember things that sounded interesting to you?" Anna asked.

Jack grinned at her, "I remember some of what Clarence recommended— The Clinic tours, both historical and art, the Italian restaurant, the park, the library, the Civic Center, and more, but I can think of other ways we can use that precious time."

Dr. Patel called for attention and invited the whole group into a large adjoining room where chairs were set up in a large circle with spaces for wheelchairs in the circle.

Here was another, smaller art collection. "Let's take time to study the art in here when this session is over," said Anna. "Maybe it has a theme too."

Dr. Patel thanked everyone for participating in her study, then briefly reviewed The Clinic's research efforts related to aging.

Krystyl (she told them to use her first name) related her personal experience with Alzheimer's through an aunt who had suffered with it for almost twenty years. Then she asked each person to introduce himself or herself and the family member patient and to tell about how long they have been dealing with Alzheimer's disease.

Jack counted as introductions proceeded: twenty patients. Six were with one of their children, two with siblings (one person had two siblings with her), and the rest with spouses. Thirteen of the twenty patients were women. So the caregivers outnumbered the patients by one.

Attendants, one for each patient, took them off to begin the testing at nine o'clock sharp. The caretakers were divided into two groups; half would move to a different, smaller room. More coffee was served. Anna said coffee is Minnesota gasoline, depended upon to keep the human motor running.

For the first time, Jack and Anna would be in different groups, each led by a social worker. Could he ask that they be kept together because they are very close? Lunch at noon meant it couldn't last forever, so he said nothing. Anna gave her fingertip wave as she left with her group.

Jack's session gave everyone a chance to share stories of experiences with Alzheimer's. Just what he and Anna had done all day yesterday. Some were funny stories and the room rang with laughter. Others were sad stories that had people reaching for their handkerchiefs. No duplication of stories and some indeed unique.

One that Jack found especially interesting was about Mary Ann, a patient who was very upset because someone was stealing her jewelry and clothing. Her daughter Karen said this was early in the illness when there were friends and family in and out of the home every day. Karen and Lucille, a good friend and next-door neighbor, set up a system to watch carefully for thievery, but found no evidence of it.

One day Mary Ann told Lucille about a two-strand pearl necklace and her favorite blue and cream-colored print dress that were taken the day before. She described each item in detail.

With that information, Lucille checked all the drawers and closets. She found the dress and there was a two-strand string of pearls in Mary Ann's jewelry box. A person would be unlikely to own two such pieces of jewelry.

Over the next few days Lucille kept talking with Mary Ann about thievery suspicions. She asked Mary Ann more questions. Sometimes Mary Ann didn't make sense, and sometimes she did. Finally, Lucille figured out that when Mary Ann looked into her large bedroom mirror, which she did often, she didn't recognize herself. Instead she saw a stranger wearing her jewelry and clothing. Mary Ann then believed that woman in the mirror had stolen them from her. They solved the problem by removing the mirror.

Each story reminded someone of another story, related or not, so the morning flew by. Promptly at noon, soup and sandwiches were delivered to the lobby. Jack met Anna there.

Nurse Johansson found them immediately to tell them that Karl and Marsha were set up for Wednesday, beginning at noon. They would meet again at lunchtime on Thursday. Other appointments needed to be rearranged slightly, so she also handed them revised schedules for the rest of the week.

"That's tomorrow!" Anna looked at Jack in a combination surprise and fear. Jack was grinning ear to ear.

Jack put his hands on Anna's shoulders, looked into her eyes and in a serious tone said, "You'll be fine. I promise."

Announcement of the beginning of the afternoon session cut through their conversation. Again the study subjects (it was hard to think of your spouse as a "study subject") were taken to testing areas. The caregivers gathered in the same large room off the lobby.

In the few minutes before everyone was settled, Jack walked around the periphery with Anna, looking at the pictures on the walls. When in the room before, they had hardly noticed anything there, but were aware of bright colors used in a few works. Most, however, were in dark, even drab colors. If there were definite objects, it was hard to find them. Certainly not representational art. If a theme united the works, it might be "other worldly" in that it was difficult to understand what the art represented. No offering of titles or any other hints existed.

Again they sat in a circle, without spaces for wheelchairs. Dr. Stanley Rosenberg, a psychologist, led the session. He first asked them to tell him their names, then tell how they had known that their loved one had serious dementia.

Then more questions. When did they know it? What did they do about it? How slowly or how quickly did they seek medical or other help? How did they cope with knowing it was probably Alzheimer's disease?

Anna said softly, "It's really hard to think of a song that fits in with all those questions."

Peter, whose mother suffered from the disease, heard Anna's question. "How about 'Make the World Go Away'? I'm a big country music fan and once heard Eddy Arnold sing that in person. Expresses my wish--take it all off my shoulders. Do and say what you used to before Alzheimer's took you away". I sing that to my mom. I'm no Eddy Arnold, but..."

"Oh, I understand," Anna gripped his hand. I feel that way too. I suppose all of us do."

Dr. Rosenberg raised his hand to quiet their talking in the group of three. Rosenberg asked Anna to share their conversation with everyone. With Peter's help, they did. That started the conversational ball rolling. Soon caregiver descriptions of their feelings poured forth. Then Rosenberg turned the topic to help for caregivers, especially in the early stages of their loved ones' illness.

Neither Jack nor Anna could believe what Rosenberg thought should be done when the disease descends. One suggestion was to write a letter to family, friends, and neighbors announcing that your loved one has dementia, possibly Alzheimer's, and telling what can be expected in the near future.

"Sounds like a greeting of bad tidings," said Jack to the laughter of the group. "And to update that writing every few months, well, I wouldn't think of it. And if I thought of it, I wouldn't do it."

Another suggestion: if the caregiver can't do outside work, ask a neighbor to help with your yard work once a week. If driving to do errands or for doctor visits is a problem, ask others to drive you.

Anna could see the letter idea as good for her sons' families, but not to anyone else. So their different two-cent pieces clinked into the ring. Jack had to hand it to Dr. R. in that he made it easy for anyone to add comments along the way. Almost everyone had comments to offer. Many liked ideas that Jack didn't like. So different strokes for different folks, he thought, and shrugged.

A sensitive discussion concerned helping children understand and relate to Alzheimer's victims. One of Rosenberg's suggestions was to use videos explaining the disease in everyday language. Charles, a man who had young children, commented, "Kids will watch anything on a TV screen. Doesn't mean they understand what they see."

Dr. R ignored that and noted that the situation is usually one of a grandparent and grandchildren. Anna then told her story of grandchildren at ages four and seven, to whom their Opa's failing mind and body had been explained. They nicknamed him "Allzees". That became "All Zs", which to them meant the end of the alphabet and the end of Opa. They were scared by that idea and the older one wouldn't write a "Z" for some time. Maybe he thought writing it would kill his grandfather.

On another visit a year later, parents and Oma offered more explanation to the children. They accepted the Zs and proceeded to make paper signs with that letter in all sizes and colors to pin to Opa's clothing. Even painted Zs on his face!

Anna noted that it was unusual for Karl not to react in some way, often a noisy, disruptive outburst. He never did that when the grandchildren were with him. She felt somehow he related to children with more patience than he showed her.

Were the grandchildren using Opa as a plaything? They remembered their earlier Opa, but the connection to that man had come unplugged. They never really connected to their new and changing Opa. To them, he was a strange object, one that talked funny, walked funny, and acted funny. Not a person, let alone their Opa, but a different kind of creature.

The children would laugh at him and that hurt Anna, not Karl. She said, "I think they put me in the same box as Karl. It's true. I'm no longer a separate person to them, just an appendage to Karl. They live on the coast and come to Minnesota rarely. That's because of their parents' discomfort."

For all the stories Anna had told, Jack had not heard about her grandchildren. Maybe she hadn't talked about them, knowing he had none. Maybe now it's not so bad to have no grandchildren. Not long ago he'd thought that would be the greatest.

Jack loved his paternal grandfather. They'd spent a lot of time together, often busy repairing things. Granddad was an expert fixer, everything from a chipped cup to a broken axle on the car. It had been fun to work with him. Granddad did the main work and talked a lot while doing it. He let Jack help and praised his contributions. When Granddad died, he grieved more and longer than when his father died.

On the topic of how the caregivers coped with their problems, the point that struck Jack was that he and Anna were the only two of the twenty-one caregivers who used no outside help for their family member or for household chores.

Some had adult day-care facilities

that accepted Alzheimer's patients. That would give anywhere from three to eight hours of free time in a day. For one family, the availability of day respite came only once a week. For some, it was available five days per week.

Others hired home aides to relieve them for one or more days per week. Some had volunteers who came to the home to help for anywhere from an hour to several hours. Some of the help consisted of just being with the patient. Others provided some housework along with being there.

A few participants chided both Jack and Anna for going it alone, saying it wasn't healthy, a bad idea, a big mistake. Neither Jack nor Anna said anything in response to the remarks. Dr. Rosenberg interrupted to say he would talk with Anna and Jack about that later and moved the group on to another topic.

At 4:00 the session ended. They only needed to wait for Marsha and Karl to be brought back. Another cup of coffee in hand, they looked at the artwork again, taking more time. "What do they have in common? It's not caregiving, for sure." Anna went from one to another of the pieces, then back.

"Maybe fantasy?" asked Jack.

"Maybe."

"Maybe we don't understand art."

Karl walked out with Ben, his attendant and another brought his chair behind them. "We've been asking Karl to keep moving this afternoon. He's done well, but is tired now." He helped Karl into his wheelchair.

Marsha came in her wheelchair. Jack asked if she had been walking much. Janine, her attendant, said that walking therapy would begin in one or two days for Marsha. So she and Karl were not on the same schedule—a surprise.

Outdoors everything gleamed in the sun. A gorgeous day—shameful to have spent it all inside the Oyam Center. "Do you feel like taking the long way back, Anna? It would be nice to get more time outside."

"Yes," replied Anna, "I'm tired of sitting so much and being in the midst of a larger group all day. A longer walk sounds wonderful."

They explored residential areas stretching away from the highway. Nice and quiet. "Anna, how about going out to dinner tonight? A restaurant meal for a change. Feel like it?"

"Sure. There are a lot of choices. Let's use my Buick. Lots of room for the wheelchairs in its trunk."

After an hour-long walk, they

stopped in their rooms to freshen up and tend to Marsha and Karl, then headed out to the little Italian restaurant Clarence had recommended.

Carlotti's lighting enticed them. Low, with lighted candles on the tables. After looking at the dozens of choices on the menu, they ordered chianti and spaghetti with meatballs for all. Karl almost went to sleep over his dinner plate and Marsha looked tired, so they did not linger.

At the door, as they prepared to use the ramp exit, who should they see but Clarence! He was in a party of six people at the main door. "Hurry, Anna, and turn your head to the left. Let's get out of here." She did as told and soon Anna drove away.

"Whew, that was a close one," Jack wiped his forehead. "I spotted Clarence coming into the restaurant with a group."

"You mean you didn't even want to say hello? It might have been safe to say hello since he was with others. I still think he's just lonely."

"No way. I take no chances with that guy. Besides, we need time to talk this evening—with each other, not Clarence. I do owe him a better thank you and if I had his address, I'd write him a thank you from California later."

Bedtime preparations for Karl and Marsha took longer than usual. Both dragged through the routine, very tired. "Where shall we put them to bed?" Jack looked quizzically at Anna.

"They put themselves together last night. Should we put them into separate beds tonight? Tonight they are even more tired than last night, so I'll bet they both sleep well wherever they're put."

"How about putting them together

again. If it's working, why change it?" Jack picked Marsha up and put her in Anna's bed. He then helped Karl get settled there too. The move met no resistance, and when Karl lay flat, he was snoring after taking about five breaths.

Jack shaved, then found nice music on the radio and cleared as much space as possible by moving the table from 116 to 114. He invited Anna to dance. The carpet did not substitute for a good wood floor, but it didn't make dancing impossible either.

Jack held her closer and she melded with him. "Anna, I love holding you." They danced together smoothly.

"It feels great to be held," Anna smiled up at him. The music stopped, the dancing stopped, and the kiss started. It was a long, lingering, luxurious kiss, mouths moving together as if still dancing to music and bodies pressing hard.

"Look, we're close like this, and for the first time, I'm not crying with my head on your shoulder. Being with you turns my body's vibrate button on and every cell does just that. You excite me."

"I may excite you. You ignite me." They laughed. "Did you know one definition of dancing is making love to music?" Jack asked. "We could turn out the lights and do 'Dancing in the Dark'. I know the tune, but not any words. Do you know the words?"

"No, afraid not. I'd be a little afraid of dancing with you in the dark right now."

"I love you, Anna." Jack's eyes searched her face, serious now. "I need you. We have the gift of precious time together. We've both worried about lost memories for so long, now you and I could make some wonderful new memories together."

"You are an inordinately attractive man, Jack." Anna said it, then hesitated. "I don't know why I said that. You are, of course, but I'm sure you don't need to be told. I mean…" She waited, then said, "I guess I'm afraid of my own feelings toward you."

"Anna, I accept your compliment. I felt a strong attraction to you from the beginning. In the first couple of hours yesterday, I knew I truly loved you. I thought I was beyond sexual arousal, but while I held you under that cafeteria table, my body showed me I wasn't."

"I think we're talking about lust. I'm susceptible to it too. The idea of adultery, however, doesn't appeal to me at all—anytime with anyone."

"I don't have a scarlet letter A to offer you, Anna. I've been totally faithful to Marsha. I love the woman she used to be. The woman she is now resembles that woman in only a few superficial ways. I promised to love her until death parts us. In many ways, my wife has left this life."

Anna held the silence for minutes. "Jack, if I were to have an affair with anyone, and you were interested in me, it would be with you. But I don't think I'm capable of having an affair. It isn't because I don't want you. I do. My value system proscribes sex before marriage in spite of what the world does today and it expects faithfulness to my marriage partner until death—the no-breathing kind of death."

Jack nodded, "I believe Marsha shared your value system. I am human. I have not felt human in a long time. As I said before: for the first time in years, I feel ALIVE. Maybe it's being with you, an attractive, intelligent woman who understands me as no one else does. Maybe it's hormones surging after being repressed so long. Who knows? I know with certainty that I feel a powerful attraction to you, all of you."

"I can't deny feeling strongly attracted to you as well."

"Sex is a basic human need, like food."

"Jack, we can't live without food, but we can last a long time without sex."

"I know that all too well. We've both lasted a long time without it."

Anna just looked at him, mute.

"I will not push you, Anna. If there is to be anything sexual between us, you must want to be my partner. I value you as a friend—my best friend. That means everything to me. You don't need to worry about anything more. I will respect your no, if that is your decision."

They moved apart and soon were settled in bed, each wishing to be with the other.

8   Anna

"You don't need to worry about anything more. I will respect your no, if that is your decision." Jack's words echoed over and over in Anna's ears.

His voice sounded calm, objective, but the look on his face betrayed his words. How to describe it? Utter dejection. Disappointment. Hurt. Raw pain. His expression belied his words. It hurt to see him.

She did not want to cause him discomfort in any way. After all he had done for her, it felt terrible. He was her best friend and she couldn't lose that. She prepared for bed and soon was settled, glad the bed was large and Karl was sleeping better. So close to Jack and now—a big gap between them. Could that gap be bridged?

Almost immediately Anna could hear Jack's deep breathing. How could he sleep when she couldn't? She wanted to sleep with Jack because of two things: Jack's attractiveness and her own long abstinence from sex.

He wanted sex. That was clear. But then, didn't all men? Most of them, anyway. Sex always sat on the front burner of male brains. Brains? Well, maybe some lower level. Men give it high priority, wherever it is.

She had said no, and thought that was clear. But—so many buts. When she said no—his face, oh how could she stand that hurt expression? He seemed to sag under an unbearable load. She couldn't turn off that image of him. He tried to hide those feelings under calm, rational words as cover.

He said I had to want to. If I said no, he would respect my no. Can't help but feel that Jack is an honorable man. That put the ball in my court. What do I do with the ball? What about my "no" left him waiting—for a different answer? What is it *I* don't understand about my "no"?

I'm lying in a comfortable bed, with no comfort. The bedside clock shows 10:00. Staring up into the dark doesn't stop my mind from twirling wildly. I know what Jack wants all right. He's been deprived and I'm handy. Couldn't be handier! From under the table to sharing time, room, spouses, everything.

Maybe that's all there is to it—just human nature or animal lust or sexual magnetism. It might mean nothing. Anna turned on her left side, facing the wall.

He's been so good to me. Considerate. Obviously likes to talk to me and be with me. Could all of that have been planned just to seduce me? No, I don't think so. And I like talking to him and being with him. I need that!

Have things changed so much since I was young? As a teenager, I heard that F word very rarely. The connotation was raw, animal sex, devoid of any love connotations. Today F-ing seems to be the favorite adjective for use with *any* noun. I have trouble with hearing this so often, but hope "this too, shall pass". Today's teens did not invent the word. We can hope they are able to wear it out with overuse.

Some people of my day recited their repertoires of dirty jokes, and I guess anyone would understand them today. Telling the jokes and acting them out weren't related though—one didn't necessarily lead to the other.

Dating in my rural Minnesota area involved doing something with someone—dancing, going to a movie, seeing a play, going to church and church activities, playing games, and even working together. "Going out" put groups of young people together. Didn't even need to have an even number of boys and girls. Drivers lucky enough to obtain use of the family vehicle for an evening or weekend afternoon would gather friends from the farms and in town. The drivers and their full loads (there were no seat belts available then, so "pack 'em in" maximized the passenger capacity) could bring a crowd to a dance in some village 30 to 50 miles away.

Couple dating began during the last two years of high school, when pairing added to the mix, but one still participated in the group "goings" as they were called. Doing things together on these dates resulted in getting to know others better.

The whole community subscribed to the common code of sexual abstinence prior to marriage, the virtue of virginity, and the importance of good judgment in choosing a mate.

Eddie, the only illegitimate child I ever knew, lived in town. He was almost 10 years younger than I, so we spent little time together. Eddie and Liz, his mother, lived in a small house in this town where she had grown up and where her parents continued to live.

Liz had been engaged to Marty Hanson almost a year. It was late 1942 when Marty was drafted into World War II. During his short time before reporting for duty, they planned their wedding for the first leave he expected—that Christmas. Instead of a leave, Marty's concentrated training led to immediate deployment in Europe to fight the Germans.

In one of the first enemy encounters there, Marty was killed. When Liz learned of his death, she knew she was pregnant. She hadn't written to tell Marty, expecting he would be home soon—she would surprise him with the news then. So Marty never knew he would have a child.

Liz and Eddie were generally accepted, although Eddie suffered a lot of schoolyard insults and they never stopped. The grounds for acceptance included patriotism.

That story is probably still told in my home community half a century later. I'm sure the moral is emphasized—no sex before marriage. Do the young people there reject that now?

Hormonal pressure being what it was then, and still is, and probably always will be, a few couples broke the code. Pregnancies resulted sometimes, followed by hurried marriages. People stigmatized these with words—shotgun wedding, "premature" babies, and haste makes babies. Reliable birth control has made a huge difference.

Other couples abstained through years-long engagements. The Great

Depression left enduring fear of poverty and loss of property in its survivors. Being able to support a wife and family ranked as the number one criterion for male marriageability.

How could I even think of extramarital sex? It violates every principle I have. Those principles came from that small rural home community. Do they apply now—in other places, among people of different backgrounds, people of different ages? They used to kill people for adultery—some countries still do.

Anyway, it's wrong. Still, I can't think of anything but adultery right now. The clock registers 11:55 pm.

Jack's face, his beautiful face, looms in my mind. The look on that face when I said no. Crestfallen, disappointed. Sleep won't come, that image holds me in an iron vise.

I really like the man a great deal. It feels wrong to refuse him. He's been my hero, my rescuer. What would have happened without him? What might still happen *with* him? He's the closest friend I've ever had. I want his friendship. I need it. I do not want to disappoint him.

Let the devil take tomorrow, but tonight I need a friend. That song must be about sex. Hadn't thought of it before, but now I could have written it.

When he wanted to hold me or kiss me, I wanted it too. Had I led him on? Does he think I've been a tease? Do I love him? Really love him? I think I do, but can that happen in a few days? Shouldn't be possible. Does falling in lust happen faster?

Well, I'm disappointed too. She made an involuntary sound and sat bolt upright. She did not want to awaken Jack, whose regular breathing accompanied her anxious thinking.

Sleep wasn't going to come quickly. She yawned repeatedly.

Some pecking sounds replaced stillness. Rain against the window. Anna crept out from under the covers and reached down, feeling for her slippers. Her night-light provided just enough light to keep from crashing into something big. Jack had brought one too. His lit the other bedroom, but gave a sliver of light here too. Pushing her feet into the slippers, she got up quietly and walked to the little table and chair by the window.

She opened the drapes part way and sat down to watch the motion of raindrops forming little rivers flowing downward on the glass. Hearing the raindrops and watching the patterns as they combined and recombined were hypnotic and soothing. Maybe they can lull me into sleepiness. I'd like the rain to wash away thoughts of Jack, at least for now.

Lightning flashed, warning of a possible storm. Stormy weather—she couldn't finish the thought because the song jumped in to interrupt. Yes, it's stormy when my man and I aren't together on what to do about love. Will it keep rainin' all the time as in the song? How can I coax the sun to shine again? It kept raining.

Rainy nights brought back memories of sitting with Clem, a high school boyfriend, in his dad's car one rainy night. They had driven to Lake Itasca after a baseball game. It was late and no one was around. A gentle rain, just like this one, had started. Clem had said the motor got wet and he couldn't start the car. Had said they would have to spend the night out there in the country with no one around. He had scared her, but it was all his idea of good fun to see what she would—or would not—do. She had made it as clear to Clem as she had to Jack that she was not someone who would fool around.

She went to check on Karl. From the open door between the rooms she could make out the shapes of the two bodies in bed there. They were sleeping spoon fashion and Karl's arm was around Marsha's waist. His face was against her hair. Both were sound asleep and looking peaceful.

How long had it been since Karl had slept with an arm around her? How many years? She wished for the old Karl. This was so weird to see him in bed with Marsha. So far there was nothing sexual between the two. Wonder what they think. Or do they just feel? What do they feel? What needs started their pairing? What did Karl need that I didn't or couldn't provide?

Should I just feel and quit working so hard at thinking? I try to understand this situation. It's temporary. That's certain. Why worry about something that will be all over soon? It's not worth it.

Anna went into the bathroom. Closing the door, she turned on the light. Maybe she could read something in there for a while to help make her sleepy. An old *Reader's Digest* lay next to the TV in the other room. Should she get it?

Looking in the mirror, Anna saw a tired, anxious face. "Why is this bothering me so much? My answer's NO and it needs to stay that way. I said that and will stick with it."

As Anna returned to the bed, the clock numbers read 2:30 am. Lying on her back again, she crossed her arms behind her head. Jack, Jack, Jack. All thoughts swirled around that man—his inordinate attractiveness. No doubt about it—It's more than physical attraction, though. He is so considerate.

He's intelligent and caring. He's helpful—He's a Godsend to me—I love him—I want him.

I know that I could not have stayed in Rochester with Karl if Jack hadn't come under that cafeteria table with me. We ought to put a marker of some kind under that table. It needs to be enshrined as a special place. How silly we must have looked. Jack was sure no one noticed us. But Clarence, that funny little man, noticed and couldn't resist making remarks about it. Saying we were engaged in "hanky-panky". I think he's more amusing than obnoxious. Jack doesn't like him at all. Anna turned on her right side and peered over the edge of the bed.

I'd like to be down there on the floor with Jack. Better, I'd like him to be here with me where it's more comfortable. I'm sleeping single in a double bed, like the song says. Down there it would be sleeping double on a single mattress. I'd love to have him hold me—just hold me.

It's wonderful to have a friend like Jack. I need him. I don't want this thing about sleeping together to get in the way of our friendship. I want him. I admit it. I do want him. In that way. Or do I? It's been so long since I've made love. I thought it was over for the rest of my life. Now here I am—just like a lovesick teenager.

Do I love Jack? Truly love him? Where could a mutual love lead us—if that is what this is? More important, does he love me or is it purely and only physical attraction? I'm confused and stressed out. Some song says that when somebody loves you, it's no good unless he loves you—all the way. Do I give up everything if I don't go all the way? What to do? The clock shows 3:30 a.m.

She played out all sorts of scenarios, worried about things like her wrinkled upper thighs, the flab roll around her waist. The numerous wrinkles on her face should signal there might be more signs of aging elsewhere on her body. Would there be a light on?

What a long night. Only one other like it—the night Erik was born. I'd been in labor since noon. At first it was exciting. The baby was coming. Our first. I called my doctor. We waited at home for the pains to be closer together. Karl didn't go to the store. He kept a log of the times and finally, we headed for the hospital at six o'clock. Suppertime. There was no supper for us that evening. Karl didn't want to be at home any longer. He wanted us to be close to all the help we could possibly need.

Time dragged its feet then too. Lots of anxiety. Would our baby be healthy? What if there were serious problems? More likely to be a happy ending. When would we know? It didn't seem bad, just excruciatingly loooooong. But there was a happy ending.

Jack stirred. He was getting up. Would he come to her? Should she say something? If so, what? Anna watched Jack move toward the bathroom. Soon he emerged and went into the next room. Anna bet he too checked their sleeping mates. Then he slipped back into his sleeping bag on the floor. Soon his slow, regular breathing showed that he slept again.

Sleep would not come to Anna, so she got up again. She started walking in a figure eight, making a loop in this bedroom, then going into the other bedroom to do the same. She needed to clear her mind. Maybe a little exercise could help her get to sleep. After what seemed like hours, Anna couldn't put one slippered foot in front of the other.

The clock advanced to 4:45. It was beginning to be light outside. Early birds were chirping in nearby trees. She closed the drapes and climbed between the sheets to toss from side to side trying to find respite. Jack occupied every thought, every moment. The clock seemed to watch her and count out the minutes. "I'm going to be a zombie for the rest of this day," she whispered to herself.

When I was young, there were three reasons to "shun" sex: detection, infection, and conception. It's different when you're a senior citizen. No fear of conception. It's not possible. Detection wouldn't matter either. At least not in this case. Infection, though, could be a real danger. I've heard that seniors have a growing rate of what we called venereal diseases or VD. Now the designation is STDs or STIs.

Could Jack be a carrier of that type of disease? From everything he said and from what he seemed, no. But what if? Should she ask him to use a condom?

Would he have one to use? Maybe asking would insult him. When I told him that Karl was the only sexual partner I've ever had and that marriage came before any sex, he didn't say, "Me too."

Could I do this with Jack? Am I ready? I remember my granddaughter's fascination with my wedding ring when she was little. She brought a friend in to look at it, saying "Come see my Granma's *ready* ring!" I liked that. A wedding ring should be a ready ring. I was ready for mine.

What would my grandchildren think if I asked them? Of course, I wouldn't do that, but I wonder. They probably think grandparents don't have sex anyway.

As teens, passion is limited to squirting organs. One can only hope that they will develop and mature to a level where they begin to understand, appreciate, and experience the depth and scope of everything that true passion has to offer. I wish that each could experience a passionate, deep, enduring, satisfying, compassionate, true love. How fortunate they would be.

I know their parents try to teach morals, but it's against the battering ram of TV, movies, and music lyrics. I'm glad I'm not a parent of youngsters today. I've shared my ideas, but can't expect them to adopt them. Probably I seem terribly old-fashioned, no matter what I say. Grandchildren have to help grandparents with computers and all the other electronic gear, so what could the old folks possibly know? There aren't many popular shows or books or music about senior sex. Maybe there should be.

I can't imagine having sex just to have sex. Love and Sex. Don't they go together? Sure, there is love without sex, maybe lots more than with it. Love of family, love of friends, love of heroes (or celebrities today).

And yes, there is sex without love. There's the dark, seamy side of sex-- prostitution, pedophilia, pornography, all that. The other person is more a target than a human being with feelings, even feelings of fear or pain, let alone love.

Sex minus love is meaningless, casual sex. Sex done for entertainment. They call it hooking up now.

Sex and love together should bring out the best of each and the best in the partners. When you love someone, you trust him. You have confidence in your lover. Then you can freely abandon inhibitions and enjoy each other. It's blending bodies and hearts. It's spiritual, life affirming, and more. I do want that. It's been so long.

It could be wonderful. But maybe it could be awful too. Is it adultery when a spouse isn't really "living" in a sexual sense? How about a spouse sleeping with someone else who he thinks is his wife? Does that free me in any way? Probably not. When is adultery not *really* adultery? Am I just looking for a justification?

Rationalizing because I want this? How much is not wanting to hurt Jack? Can I change a no to a yes? What to do? I really can't make a decision. Or do I just not want to. Ah, the song...

First you say you do
and then you don't.
You're undecided now
so what are you gonna do?

The song repeated and repeated in my mind until the alarm went off at 7:30 am. What a night. How can I get through this day?

9   Jack

Jack awoke to the buzz of the alarm. For the way he felt, it should have sounded like a foghorn. He laughed at himself sardonically. He tried to focus on his surroundings, but to no avail. It was as if a platoon of spiders had woven an impenetrable web over his eyes. Or, he mused, which wasn't clear—his mind or his eyes?

He stretched his arms toward the ceiling, then sat up cross-legged on the floor mattress and stretched some more. Feeling ready to face the day's challenges, he made a trip to the bathroom. There he danced as he brushed his teeth while standing on the cold tiles that shocked his bare feet.

A glance into the adjoining room showed Marsha and Karl still sound asleep. Peacefully, thank God.

Turning, he noticed Anna sitting by the window. She looked awful. Pale face, red eyes, and sagging posture. In panic, he rushed to her.

"Anna, my precious, are you OK? Are you ill? What's wrong?" He knelt in front of her chair and held her shoulders to see if a closer look might reassure him. It didn't. "What is it? Please talk to me!" Her face showed no expression. He cradled her in his arms, feeling the coldness of her body.

"I'm OK, or at least not ill. I just spent a sleepless night."

"I had a good night's sleep, and you needed it more than I. I'm so sorry you had a bad night." He hugged her tight and rubbed her back.

In the motel breakfast room, Anna ate a single roll and drank two cups of coffee. Jack ate everything the HighWay had to offer. Why was he eating so much? Maybe stress eating? Was he gathering strength to face rejection? He thought their partners ate unusually well and quickly.

"I spent the night thinking instead of sleeping, Jack. Even with two cups of coffee for starter fluid, I'm afraid it's going to be a long day.

"Since we're through with breakfast early, could we walk through the residential streets instead of by the highway? That won't be so noisy and we can talk."

After they turned the corner to walk away from the motel he said, "OK Anna, now tell me why you had a sleepless night."

"I thought of you and the last part of our conversation last night. I felt terribly conflicted. I don't want to do anything that would be wrong for me, for Karl, or for our marriage. Yet I agree with you that the 'marriage' partnership joins caregiver and care receiver. There's almost no positive emotional contact between us, and too much negative. Is my partner 'dead' as you describe? I thought about that for a long time.

"Then I thought of the song words, 'Let the devil take tomorrow, but tonight I need a friend.' I need you, Jack. But I didn't feel ready to make a change from friend to lover. You are the best and most important friend I've ever had."

"Anna, I think we would add another dimension to our friendship that would enhance it, not damage it."

"I hear you. I feel nervous and excited at the same time. Even without a moment of sleep, I am wide awake now. Totally awake. Maybe it's the caffeine kicking in. I fought with myself, but came to a decision that I think is right. Right for me. Right for now. Right for both of us. It may be wrong in other ways, but my decision is made. Coming to it was agonizing, but once there, I'm relieved and comfortable with it. I keep telling myself this is only temporary, a little slice of life for both of us. A few days to experience love."

Anna said nothing more for almost two blocks. Jack let the silence remain undisturbed. Was she trying to soften her rejection? He couldn't confidently translate her words into a yes or a no. Just before reaching their destination, Anna stopped suddenly, turned to Jack and announced in a firm voice, "Jack, I'm ready to earn my scarlet A. Do they come in pairs?"

Jack reached for her. He was ecstatic. He kissed her—a long one. Her face was soft, a slight smile on her lips. He cleared his throat, then said slowly, "I love you, Anna."

"I love you too, my dear Jack."

His eyes misted and he pulled her even closer, "The time we've been together can be measured best in hours, but you are a permanent part of me. I'm incomplete without you. I feel I've known you my entire life. I want you, Anna. I want you forever."

"Forever might be out of reach. We have now. Only now. What's left of one week. I want you for now. We can't count on long term for so many reasons. You know them as well as I do."

They finished the last short part of the walk silently, walking briskly. As they pushed their partners up the rampway to the Oyam Center, Jack hoped Anna was truly ready for this new experience between them in addition to the new experiences of the Alzheimer's study.

Yes, their friendship was as comfortable as old worn shoes, but for him it was closely related to his excitement at being with this warm, sweet, attractive woman.

The same array of breakfast offerings adorned the lobby table, with coffee, of course. Now Anna ate more than she had earlier. He was so full from breakfast that he could only drink some juice. Both Marsha and Karl enjoyed some doughnut holes. Even those had to be broken into eight pieces for Marsha. Karl could chew a whole one with ease. He ate three of them.

Janine and Ben came for their charges and spirited them away. Jack and Anna joined the caregivers group. They sat together and held hands. His other hand caressed the top of her hand. Even their feet reached for each other. Anna rubbed her foot against the back of his ankle. Could she know how this excited him?

There was a program going on, but neither was aware of the topic or even the people surrounding them. Noon seemed so far away. He did not want to sit here. Could they leave early? If so, right away? Anna looked ill enough to make leaving plausible. He whispered to Anna, "Shall we play hooky and leave now? We know that Marsha and Karl are taken care of from now on."

"What about lunch time?" Anna whispered back, "This session will be our last meeting with the caregivers program before the sleep study begins."

"If it's OK with you, I'll just say you aren't feeling well and need to go back to the motel. That's no lie. My poor dear one, you need rest badly."

"It's OK with me. I'm not getting anything out of the program today." They left together quietly. Jack told the receptionist their reason for leaving and said they'd be back tomorrow at noon.

Taking Anna's arm, he led her to a comfortable chair. "Anna, please wait here. I'll drive you back to the motel."

She protested, but not vigorously. He actually ran part of the way back and danced the rest. In a very few minutes they were in their motel "duplex".

"Anna, I'm worried about you. You must get some sleep. I'll draw all the drapes and put out the Do Not Disturb sign."

"During those few minutes at the Center while waiting for you, I thought about being a care receiver. Jack, you are my caregiver today. I feel cared about, protected, and loved. It's a warm, wonderful feeling. Do you suppose Karl and Marsha have those feelings sometimes or somehow?"

"I hadn't thought about it quite that way. I think a relationship exists, but it's a very complex one. One I don't really understand, let alone what Marsha feels. What I do know is that I care about and love you. I will do anything I can for you."

"I know you do, Jack, and you know I feel exactly the same. Thank you."

He kissed her, then said he'd tuck her in. Anna changed back to her nightgown and gratefully slid between the sheets of her bed. She shivered.

"Cold, Anna?"

"Just a chill. Don't know why."

"I can offer some assistance for that. I'll hold you close and we can sleep together."

"I don't..."

"Anna, I mean sleep, just sleep, not *that* kind of sleep together, just the eyes closed, deep breathing kind. I'll help keep you warm." He got in bed next to her facing her back and put his arm around her, nestling with her as close as two spoons in the silverware drawer.

"You have a wonderfully warm body. Thank you. It feels good to be held like this."

She was asleep almost before she finished her sentence. Jack stayed a while, relishing the feel of this woman so close to him. So glad the Center was conducting a sleep study. After an hour, he got up to read a book he'd brought.

Not wanting to turn on a light, which might disturb Anna, he took this new history about World War II on the home front out to the lobby to read it. He was born just before that war began and could remember little from his early childhood, so this book should be interesting.

He poured himself a cup of coffee from the ever-full pot in the lobby and sat down to enjoy it while reading. When his cup was empty, he hadn't read two pages. Thinking about Anna, thrilling to the thoughts. More important, he wanted to be back in the same room with her. It wouldn't be good for her to awaken and find him gone.

Entering quiet, dark room 116, it was clear Anna slept on. Wonder how long she might sleep. Definitely don't want to awaken her. Let her sleep so long as she needs. He took his book into the bathroom, closed the door and turned on the light. There he sat and read with interest, if not comfort.

He took a break to shave again. Then back to the dark room. He could have closed the door between 114 and 116 and had a room to himself. Why hadn't he done that? Same reason he couldn't sit in the lobby—too far from Anna.

Anna stirred at a little after three o'clock. "Jack, are you here?"

"Yes, my love. Right here." He turned on a lamp.

She sat up and looked at the clock. "Oh, my, I slept for hours!"

Jack opened the drapes to let warm sunshine enter. Looking at Anna in the full light of day he was relieved that she looked well again. The haggard, gray look of this morning was gone. "I hope you feel as good as you look."

"I'll have to go look in the mirror to check." She headed for the bathroom. "Is there any reason to get dressed again?" she called out to Jack.

"I suggest we go the other direction. As far as nature lets us. Birthday suits are the order of the day."

"OK." Anna soon emerged with her nightgown draped over one shoulder.

Jack hurriedly expelled himself from his clothes and moved toward her. How great to hold her. "You always dress so well, but I think you look best right now. You are beautiful."

"We're going to have spectators at the windows soon," Anna said, nodding toward the big picture window. Jack closed the drapes.

They made love with fiery passion, energetically crescendoing through moves that took their breath away and brought cries of pleasure. They sank back to rest in each other's arms. Before long, a second wave of longing swept over him. This time slow, deliberate, leisurely in tempo. Just as satisfying.

They headed for the shower together. What fun! Scrubbing each other's backs, moving together and laughing at the slipperiness the soap provided between their skins. Ending by drying each other off with towels. He couldn't help but think of the contrast to showering with Marsha where his job description focused on keeping her vertical and safe from harm more than cleaning her body.

"A question, Jack. The song 'After the Loving' says I'm still in love with you. Do you still love me after the loving? " Anna immediately felt that question shouldn't have been asked. Yet she wanted his answer. Those darn songs.

"Of course. I loved you before, during, and after—and forever after too. Now the big question. What do we do about dinner? We could go out anywhere in town or we could order a pizza."

"I've lost any desire to show you the town highlights that I know, let alone Clarence's list. I only want to be with you."

"I agree. Whatever I do, I want it to be with you. And I still want forever."

"Jack, I can do without food. I can't do without you. You fulfill me." Then she laughed, "You do indeed *full fill* me."

"You wonderful woman, you." He hugged her. "How about pizza? Or something else to order for here?"

"Pizza would be great. I like black olives and green peppers on mine."

Jack picked up the phone. "That you shall have."

10   Anna

Thursday morning, her fourth morning to wake up here. What time is it? I don't want to be anywhere but right here, next to Jack—forever. How I regret those hours wasted sleeping yesterday. We need to get to the Oyam Center, but not for a while. At twelve noon instead of twelve midnight, the beautiful coach will turn back into a pumpkin. The Prince and Cinderella have to return to reality. Just remember, the Prince kept looking until he found Cinderella again. Will we ever be together after this week? If that's a no, please don't let this week ever end.

She slipped out of bed quietly, but Jack awakened. "Good morning," he said sleepily.

"I didn't mean to wake you. Go back to sleep, I'll be here."

"No way, we have precious hours to spend together, and I want to be awake. You brought me back to life and I want to live it." He got up and embraced her. "You look better than ever. How are you feeling?"

"I'm a little bit sore and a lot happy." He frowned and looked puzzled. "No, no real problem." She shouldn't have said anything. The last thing she wanted was to complain and deter him. "I should have used something to lubricate a bit more. I'm sorry, it just goes with being post-menopausal, I'm afraid."

He looked thoughtful, then said, "I think I have something in my toiletries bag that will work. Willing to try it?"

From the circle of his warm arms, she answered, "Were you a Boy Scout? You always seem prepared. First the air mattress and now... Sure, let's try it."

"Yesterday was so great, Anna. We must have an encore. How about now?"

"Give me a few minutes of bathroom time. I need to exchange my morning mouth for a fresher one."

"OK, give me five too. I'll shave and be right back. Nice to have two bathrooms."

In less than five minutes, they emerged and were clamped in each other's arms, passionately kissing. She didn't think their lovemaking could be any better and knew it would be wonderful even at levels well below yesterday's, but you don't get better than perfection. Their loving set a whole new higher standard for perfection.

Afterward, lying in bed, they talked. "What might have happened had we met when we were young?" Jack asked.

"Well, what are the chances that we could have met earlier? You lived in California all your life and I was growing up on a farm in Minnesota. How could we possibly have seen each other?"

"Just suppose we had, Anna. Suppose we met as young single adults."

"Well, had I just seen you, I would have been attracted to your smile first. When I saw you interacting with people, assuming Clarence wasn't around, of course, I would have seen a thoughtful, considerate, intelligent man with a nice sense of humor. How could I help but want to know you better?"

"Maybe it took me decades to become the person you think you saw. You might have found me a smart aleck, an offensive guy."

"Maybe, but I bet that your basic goodness always shone though." She hugged him.

"I see a lovely blonde maiden with the same traits you described. She may have been very shy and hard to get to know, but I would have tried my darndest."

"I want to believe in second chances, in a second life after this one. Because this beginning makes me want to experience the next parts all the way through to a happy ending." Anna lowered her head, afraid she had said too much. He knew as well as she that they were dealing with one week, not her fantasies.

Jack stroked her cheek, "I want all that. The happy ending would be guaranteed. Now we each have our obligations."

She looked at her watch, startled. "Jack, it's a quarter to twelve! I haven't paid any attention to time."

"We can make it. Let's get dressed and I'll drive us. Are you starving? I haven't even thought about breakfast. Good thing they furnish lunches. We'll clean our plates today, no matter what they offer."

"I'll miss our walk, but driving is a good way to save time, Jack. Bet I can be ready in less than three minutes." Anna dressed as she talked, "I don't like to be late, especially after playing hooky from our sessions this morning and almost all of yesterday."

In the car, Jack said that the caregivers program was secondary; they really wanted the tests on the patients and were simply giving them an opportunity to talk to others in like situations. She thought they recognized the needs of the caregivers and focused on them equally.

As they entered Oyam, the receptionist caught Jack's attention and motioned to him to come to her desk. Anna went with him.

"Dr. Rosenberg would like to talk with both of you. Would 2:30 be all right? That's the planned afternoon coffee break and you could meet him here at my desk."

"Fine for me," said Anna hesitantly, looking at Jack to see what he would say. He just nodded.

Janine and Ben brought Marsha and Karl into the room, each walking. Ben said they'd walked for about half an hour this morning. Their wheelchairs soon appeared in the lobby to use during lunch and for their afternoon sessions.

Vegetable soup, a chicken salad, and a lemon custard dessert made up for the missed breakfast. Jack patted his stomach, "That was a great lunch!"

Anna wanted to look around at the artwork again after eating. "I don't get a feeling about these as I do for the works in the lobby. Those I feel. Every one shows or tells me something about caregiving. These baffle me."

"We could ask someone what they're about." Jack suggested.

"Not yet, I want to compare them with each other some more. I can't see any obvious theme, so what might they represent?" She walked over to look closely at one of the especially dark pictures.

Marsha and Karl were taken off and they went into the caregivers' meeting room.

Lydia, one of the spouse caregivers, asked how Anna was feeling. "I saw you leave yesterday and worried about you."

Anna assured her that she was well now. Dr. Whitson, a white-haired, gentle-looking, somewhat rotund fellow announced the afternoon topic: dealing with the agitated patient.

Anna needed this session: Karl spent more time in agitation than a washing machine. Whitson said anger is very common, resulting from frustration, fear, or tension. Sometimes the reaction is extreme, perhaps the result of feeling insecure, of being ignored, belittled, or reprimanded. He emphasized that the caregiver can help limit the reaction.

As others shared their experiences and their attempts to handle situations of agitated loved ones, Anna shared her stories and focused on what was said, hoping it could help her in dealing with Karl.

Whitson stressed staying calm. Anna thought he made it sound easy, but let him try it during a bad situation. Very difficult. Sometimes she worked to calm Karl for a long time only to find Karl escalating his upset behavior. One of Whitson's rules: don't question or argue. Anna learned that long ago. Does no good—can make things worse.

She did many of the things suggested. She often massaged his shoulders or back and held his hands. Anna shared her experiences with playing or singing music to calm Karl. Others played music the patient enjoyed, especially slower, softer pieces and found it helped a lot. So it wasn't just because Karl was a musician. Anna didn't know why she hadn't appreciated the universal pull of music before this week.

A rule to never respond with physical force got a lot of emphasis. That never occurred as an option for Anna. Karl, normal or deranged, could overpower her physically and her own physical condition rated high. He's just much stronger.

Whitson taught them the five Rs about agitation: Remain calm, Respond to feelings, Reassure the person, Remove yourself, and Return later. She could memorize that list with the fingers on one hand. Could be helpful.

When the coffee was brought in at 2:20, the meeting broke. As they waited for a cup, Jack said he hadn't gotten much out of the session. He'd spent time watching the seconds change on his watch. Anna could see why. Agitation had never been a problem with Marsha. Her few spells of anxiety faded into their past.

Jack told Anna he'd been wondering why Dr. R wanted to meet with them. Coffee cups in hand, they walked out to the reception desk. Dr. Rosenberg waited for them there. After handshakes, he led them to his office on the second floor. He sat in an easy chair and they sat side by side facing him in comfortable armchairs. No hiding behind a desk for this man, thought Anna.

"I've noticed a strong affection between the two of you." The first thing out of his mouth! What caught his attention?

Jack went on the defensive, voice growling, "I don't know what you mean."

"I don't need my professional degree to see that you two have special feelings for each other. They say the world loves lovers. I'm sure others have noticed as well."

Jack's mouth was open to protest again, when Dr. Rosenberg's telephone rang. He excused himself, promising to be back shortly.

Anna could see Jack's taut jaw line. "He's nothing but Clarence with a doctor title! Our relationship is none of his business. I'm tempted to just go back to the meeting even if it bores the hell out of me."

Anna rose and stood behind him, rubbing his shoulders, "Jack, I understand how you feel. It may seem nosy to us, but I think he has a concern.

We don't know why he does, but I think that's why we're here."

Jack frowned and pounded his fist on the chair arm. "I didn't like others scolding us about being lone rangers, but I mind this guy's butting into our affairs even more. I don't think he could improve on the care I give Marsha."

Anna sat again, turned to face Jack, and held both of his hands, "I'm sorry this is hitting you all wrong. No one wants you to be hurt, most of all me, but I feel it would be good to let Dr. R. talk with us. Let's see what he has in mind."

Rosenberg came back, apologized for his brief absence, then switched topics, noting that others had chided them for not having outside help in caring for their loved ones. He wanted to discuss this with them. He said he cared about the caregiver, and if the caregiver isn't taken care of, the loved one suffers, but he believed the caregiver suffers more.

Dr. R. explored with Anna and Jack their motivations for going it alone. Both felt that the responsibility for spouse care belonged to them, not to anyone else. Further they felt they could handle it alone. With a little probing by Dr. R., they acknowledged a strong wish to stay independent. Did that mean they did not want to depend on anyone but themselves? To the end? What different ends might there be?

He talked to them about losing normal social contacts and how isolation can be harmful. Anna wanted to hum the music to 'Everybody Needs Somebody Sometime'. Rosenberg had even looked up support groups in each of their home areas and recommended they follow up to try these options. He felt day care for as little as a few hours each week could make a big and positive difference for them.

Jack flicked the chip off his shoulder after talking with Dr. R. only a short time. He even asked a number of questions. Eventually they could see that their style of solo care engendered loneliness in isolation. Dr. R. smoothly suggested that with so much in common in their home situations and having no one else to share their problems, they must find great comfort in getting to know each other well.

Anna wondered if that insight meant their relationship came only because of their isolation or loneliness and frustration as do-it-yourself caregivers. Maybe they just needed someone or anyone to care about them. It would be nice to have "Someone to Watch Over Me". She hummed the song, striving to remember some words. So their feelings might be a reaction to the situation, not love at all? She didn't want to talk about it now. Better later with Jack alone.

They were so involved in talking that it was startling to hear the signal indicating the sessions were over. Anna and Jack stood to go. Rosenberg put an arm around each of them and said, "You have something precious, take good care of it." Then he escorted them to the door.

Outside the door, Anna and Jack looked at each other in surprise. Jack said, "We don't have to look far for more things to talk about."

11   Jack

Jack and Anna picked up their conversation from the Oyam and opened it again in the evening at the little table in their room. Karl and Marsha were settled and seemed happy just to be together, so peace and quiet prevailed.

"So many challenges for us, physical, mental, emotional." Anna sighed and slumped in her chair.

"Anna, I think Dr. R. isolated the problem of isolation for us neatly. For me, I believe isolation hurts the most."

Anna rubbed her fingers, thinking, then said, "I live near the middle of our continent, about as far from an ocean in any direction as you could get. Still I often feel shipwrecked with Karl on an island. We don't have real relationships with anyone any more, not our friends, not our sons. I've lost who I am. I am the woman who lives with the weirdo. The few interactions with others are so superficial, so meaningless."

"I know, I know." Jack held her hand, "At our house, there is a third figure who lives with us. He's the Grim Reaper. Always standing nearby. He's so familiar that I call him GR, but I say it as a growl, grrrrrr, in his direction. We live with death standing in the corner. Always near."

"I don't have an image like yours, Jack, but we too live close to death. I try not to think about it too much."

"I probably think about it too much. Sometimes GR plays with us, lifting his scythe, ready to strike. Like the time Marsha had pneumonia or when she fell in the bathroom and was unconscious for several minutes."

Jack dropped his head into his hands briefly, "But then GR withdrew his weapon. I think he was pleased to be toying with me. He retreated to his corner to watch us go on, waiting, waiting, sometimes wishing."

Anna rose to put her arms around him from the back and lay her head close to his. "Jack, this sounds like depression. I'm so sorry. I truly understand." She stroked him as she continued, "Once many years ago I went to a talk by a Minnesota-born artist, Peggy Heddleson. She displayed a great number of felt creations--colorful, beautiful things. My favorite of all that I saw said 'Oh, the comfort of being fully understood'. I've never forgotten that banner and that thought."

"I like that thought too, Anna. We fully understand each other and that makes life more than comfortable. It is my salvation."

"Maybe love means full understanding. When we deal with our spouses now, understanding isn't there for either partner. Such a contrast between my understanding of you and my understanding of Karl."

The next morning they planned breakfast in the lobby. Karl finished quickly and Anna said she'd like to use the extra time to go back to the room to do some sewing. A button had detached from her jacket and she wanted to sew it back on before it got lost.

"We'll be a while, Anna. Coming out here when you're ready?"

"Sure. See you in a little while. Have to find my travel sewing kit." She left, taking Karl with her.

Having heard they liked oatmeal, the HighWay now provided the instant form. Jack thanked the clerk. He'd meant to go out to buy some, but it didn't get done.

Clarence came bouncing into the lobby. He obviously knew the time for the breakfast service. He pulled up a chair to the table where Jack was spooning oatmeal into Marsha's baby-bird mouth.

"So, Jack, how's zit goin'?"

"We're kept pretty busy with this Alzheimer's study, as we expected."

"Wanted to check in with ya. My friend switched shift and works nights now at the desk here. He's long gone. Where's Anna and her wheelie?"

Breathing a heavy sigh covering his irritation, Jack said, "Anna had some sewing chore she wanted to do. So she's in their room." He continued to scrape oatmeal from the almost empty bowl, patiently waiting for Marsha to swallow each tiny serving.

Clarence didn't offer Jack an attractive alternative. It was very quiet except for the sounds Kyalene, the new morning desk clerk, made as she prepared fresh coffee and rearranged the food offerings at the counter behind them.

Clarence watched silently for a long time, then asked, "Poor guy, ya do this feeding over and over, morning after morning. Do ya ever want to put rat poison in her oatmeal?"

Jack startled, then looked straight at Clarence and said firmly, "Of course, Clarence, I think about that all the time."

While Jack gently wiped her face and put a sweater around Marsha, nothing more was said, and before long Clarence wandered out of the motel. Anna brought Karl in his chair and announced they were ready to walk to the Oyam Center.

Kyalene called, "Mrs. Schmidt, I have a question about your credit card. Could you come to the desk for just a minute?"

Anna approached the desk and Jack wheeled Marsha just outside to wait for the Schmidts.

"This isn't about a credit card, Mrs. Schmidt. I just heard a conversation that is troubling me."

"What, Kyalene? Someone talking about me?"

"No, no, it's not about you. Clarence and Jack were talking and Clarence asked Jack if he'd thought of putting rat poison in his wife's oatmeal."

Anna raised both hands in horror, "Oh, my God, Kyalene. That couldn't be."

"That's what he said. I swear it. Then, even worse, Jack said he did think of that, said he thought about it all the time!"

"Kyalene, that is too farfetched to be taken seriously. They were making some kind of joke. You can be sure

Marsha won't be poisoned by anyone. Just forget it."

"Thank you Mrs. Schmidt. I feel so relieved. I'm so glad to have the chance to talk with you right away. I didn't know what to do."

"You just have a good day now, Kyalene. I'm glad that you have the day shift now. It's a beautiful day to be here. Everything is OK, I assure you." Anna shook her head as she turned away. What an excitable young woman. Probably watched too many crime shows on TV.

12   Anna

The morning session for caregivers focused on doctor-patient relationships. Anna thought it interesting. She realized her major contacts were with medical people. She never minded taking Karl to the doctors. That was part of taking good care of him. So her social life was conducted in medical waiting rooms and with medical people. The only other life was the life between appointments and that was less interesting than the appointments.

Jack was less positive. He whispered to Anna, "I'm always hoping they can improve things for Marsha, but nothing has worked so far. After her Monday physical, Dr. Osowski prescribed an anti-depressant. I had it filled right away and she's taken one a day, but I can see no difference."

"Don't you think it a little too early to judge what help it might be?" Anna didn't really want to get into meds and the hopes that were swallowed along with the pills.

Anna abruptly elbowed Jack. Their loud whispering didn't please those around them who looked at them disapprovingly.

"You know, Anna," Jack continued, leaning closer to her so she could hear the softer whisper he adopted. "I think doctors in general don't think Alzheimer's patients worth their precious time. They prescribe something because they think we caregivers will feel they are trying to help, but they know it's hopeless. They're just offering a pacifier."

"Everything has pluses and minuses. Karl's had side effects with things that seemed to help as well as some that didn't. And yes, I do feel better when something, anything, is being done for him."

Jack twisted in his chair, frowning, "Researchers keep trying to find something that will reverse Alzheimer's, or better, prevent it. For now, though, they're just trying to slow its progress. Doctors say we could try this or that, but I don't think they have confidence in what they're offering."

"Jack, the doctors get discouraged too. We each worry about one patient, our loved one, but they deal with dozens and how many have been cured?"

"OK. Anyway, it's almost lunch time." Jack folded his arms over his chest, prepared to wait out the last 20 minutes of the program without saying anything more.

As they entered the lobby for lunch, Anna enthusiastically noted gratin savoyard on the menu. "I love that rich, creamy soup. I hope they have those tiny bread loaves with it."

As Janine wheeled Marsha into the lobby, Jack took a look at her and hurried over. Anna followed Jack to Marsha's wheelchair. "What's wrong, Sweetheart?" His questioning gaze to Janine met a worried frown.

"She's been holding her stomach and just now she started retching, as though she's going to hurl. Did she seem well this morning? Did she have something different to eat this morning?"

Marsha went beyond retching. She leaned forward and expelled liquid with lumps of partially digested oatmeal into her lap. Jack stared. He stroked the back of Marsha's neck while Janine held a towel in front of her to catch any more vomit.

Anna's internal alarm bells clanged. She grabbed Jack's arm. "This morning Kyalene at the motel heard you and Clarence talking about poisoning Marsha's oatmeal. I couldn't believe anything like that until…" She looked at Marsha's continued gasping and gagging.

Jack stared at Anna, "Something caused this. Could it be Clarence?"

"No way to know now, but some poisons act fast. We've got to do something."

"I'm staying with Marsha. Go to the secretary over there and tell her what it might be. Ask her to call 911 or whatever they call here for emergencies."

Anna rushed over to the staff desk. "Please, call for medical help. There may be a case of poisoning."

"What? Oh, Mrs. Rutherford over there? She does look ill."

"Please, get help. I think she's been poisoned." The woman called immediately, two calls in fact.

Soon a guard was at Anna's elbow. "I'm Oyam security. We need to talk. Come with me." Anna followed him to a small room that served as a coat closet in winter. "Now tell me why you think this is a poisoning."

Anna related what Kyalene had told her. She identified Jack for the man by pointing him out from the door.

"Where could Clarence be located?" the guard asked Anna. She gave him what she knew. He hung around The Clinic for hours every day and lived in the city. The guard made some phone calls.

When an ambulance whisked Marsha away to The Clinic's emergency room, the guard detained Jack, saying people were coming to ask him a few questions. He also asked Jack about how to find Clarence. Jack described the way Clarence dressed and the guard said he had seen him when he'd been on duty at the main building.

Two police officers appeared, a man and a woman. The woman asked that everyone return to the conference room except Jack and Anna. Ben, Karl's attendant, appeared and took him back to the research labs earlier than needed. Anna tried to signal her appreciation for his thoughtfulness.

Anna told her story to the officers and they called the HighWay to see if Kyalene was still on duty. Finding that she was, the woman officer left to interrogate her.

Could Jack have tried to poison Marsha? They had talked about sometimes wishing death would come, but...? What about Clarence? Jack had never liked the man, but Anna thought Clarence always tried hard to be helpful. Is it possible he would poison Marsha to "help" Jack? No, no, no, nothing made any sense. Anna's head was pounding with a headache. "What a mess. Please, God, help us deal with it." She closed her eyes and put her head back.

Anna repeated her story to another man who was a detective with the police department. She heard him say something about arresting both of them as suspects. "Sir, I know that neither of these men would harm anyone. I don't understand..."

"Ma'am, it's our job to investigate. Your information has been helpful and we appreciate your coming forward. We'll take it from here, so you don't need to worry."

Thus excused, Anna looked for Jack. He was sitting between the police officer and another man in a suit. They were firing questions at him. Poor Jack, he looked so confused. "Look, I must go to my wife. She's sick and I need to be with her. The paramedic said they were taking her to the emergency room. Please take me there. Right away."

Anna saw the phones come out of pockets again as more calls were made. "Your wife's OK. They pumped her stomach. I'll have someone take you there in a little while. You can't stay long. Then they may take you downtown."

"Downtown? Why would I want to go downtown?" Jack looked at the speaker incredulously.

"We'll see. Maybe they'll bring you back here. Your wife could be held at the hospital for observation."

Jack stood up and put his face close to the officer's, "Look, if it were your wife who was ill, you'd want to be with her, wouldn't you? Well, I need to be with mine!" Jack spoke through gritted teeth.

Anna came to his side and put her hand on his arm. "Oh, Anna, I'm glad you are here. These people are driving me crazy. I need to go to Marsha. Wish we had driven over this morning. I don't even know where their emergency room is. You'd think they would help by taking me there."

"I'm so sorry, Jack. This is a terrible situation. Let's sit over here for now." She pointed to chairs in the nearest corner.

After almost an hour, a call came in and the detective called them all together to report. "That was the ER doctor. Marsha's stomach contents are negative for a poison. They think her new prescription medication might have caused her nausea.

"We are questioning Clarence and will let him know all is well. Sorry for the inconvenience, but you understand that your safety is always our concern." Off went the policemen, the man in the suit, and even the security guard. Anna and Jack went back to their seats.

Jack sat back wearily. "I can't believe this happened. I'm just getting the picture. Kyalene believed both Clarence and I might be planning to poison Marsha. So she alerted you. You pooh-poohed that, but then Marsha was sick and vomiting, so the poison idea seemed a possibility."

"Yes, that's it. Now I feel foolish for having raised the alarm, but I felt I had to."

"I understand. I shouldn't have said anything to Clarence when he asked if I'd thought of poisoning her oatmeal. I just wanted him to shut up. And he did, come to think of it. He left."

"I have a horrible headache. I'd like to take the rest of the afternoon off and go back to the HighWay." Anna massaged her forehead with her fingers.

"I surely won't get anything out of our discussions now."

"We'll go there too if they release Marsha. Otherwise, I'll drive to the hospital to see Marsha. Poor baby went through all that with strangers. I should have been there for her."

"This really disrupted the program today. I'll bet this becomes a story spread around here. Wonder if people will laugh about it or what."

"Can't imagine anyone thinking it funny."

Anna was almost asleep on her motel bed when she heard Jack talking as he came into the adjoining room with Marsha. "We'll just take a nap now. I brought some milk. The nurse said it would be good for you."

13   Jack

Jack got Marsha into clothes that didn't smell of vomit and made her comfortable sitting up in bed. She seemed back to normal. He'd never forget this day! Clarence was trouble any time, but this topped anything. His own careless remark rang in his mind. Why had he said it? So stupid. Pure coincidence that the desk clerk overheard it. She shared her concern with Anna and a couple of hours after that, Marsha was sick. Nausea as a side effect of medication happened sometimes, but none of us thought along those lines because of my one uncalled-for sentence.

Relief waved through his body again thinking of what could have been. Or could it? Zero chance of any one of us poisoning another person? He had to smile: if Clarence were poisoned, he'd have to be a suspect. He really didn't like the man. Suspicions once raised die a slow death and these deserved a quick execution. Think about something else.

Anna came back from the Oyam with Karl. Her headache had eased, so she decided to walk over instead of drive. She said it helped to walk off the tension. Poor Anna. Had she thought he might have poisoned Marsha? Even for a moment had she given that thought a place in her mind? Might *she* want to eliminate one of his obligations? He hadn't given that a thought, but now it made as much nonsense as anything else today. Maybe he should take up writing detective stories. Today had everything needed for plotting one.

"Jack, you OK? You're awfully quiet," Anna asked. "I'm not hungry, but I know Karl needs some food soon. What about you?"

"I'm not hungry either and Marsha needs to be fed carefully for a while. I'm to cut her medication dose in half for a week, then up it again if no problems. Always complications, aren't there?"

"I think I'll drive to that big grocery store to buy some ready-to-eat food for Karl and me. May I get some things for you?"

Jack asked for soup and bread for himself and Marsha. Anna left Karl in the room.

Alone with his thoughts again, Jack pondered the end of the week. It seemed closer to the end of the world to him. What a week. What a day. The good, the bad, and the ugly. Is that a song or maybe a movie? The good means Anna. The bad fits Clarence, and I can't think of anyone ugly.

How will it be back in Thousand Oaks? Things have changed. I've changed. The week gave me good information on helping Marsha and myself in new and different ways. The diagnosis of depression seems right. That condition might be there, nesting spoon fashion with the Alzheimer's. Wonder why our California doctor didn't follow up on it. Another doctor diagnosed it years ago and treated it with medication. Guess they thought it was cured forever. Wrong. Hope the medicine makes a difference now. I'd like to see some responsiveness from Marsha. Maybe I've neglected her--not understanding that she might be seriously depressed. Hell, anyone who's seriously ill has reason to be depressed.

Going home again. Without Anna it will be hard. Very hard. I love her. I need her. I know we can't be together, at least not now. This week will fade and fall like the large breasts in that poem or Marsha's prom corsage. It's not meant to be more than one wonderful week of loving. Will she write to me? Call? She has a family, sons, grandchildren. They might come more often if she can tell them how much it means to her. I don't have that.

He looked at a brochure he'd picked up on Monday at the big building. It described an apartment building adjoining The Clinic. That could be a way to stay here if Anna could do that too. Might be justified if medical care were a constant for Marsha, but it's not. They'd like to see the Alzheimer's patients in a year. Another study to follow up on this group. They said it would be only three or four days next year since the background studies are done. Same time next year? Song or movie? He didn't know.

Jack felt so down today. Like he had when he came. He and Marsha both suffered depression. Really not much different, but for different reasons. He hadn't known his own feelings. Anna lifted him up and today even her spirits are down like mine, but not as far down.

He felt so low that he'd have to look up to see bottom.

I'd like to run away from home. Haven't said that since teen years. Didn't mean it then. Do now. I'd take Anna and we'd go someplace quiet and peaceful. Ah, the fantasies.

One of the mystery art pieces came to him—a jumble of shapes and colors, all swirling around the center. That's a picture of my thoughts.

Jack straightened, "I got the picture—the real picture. All those are works by Alzheimer's patients!" We couldn't figure out the theme, but I'll bet that's it. Maybe it's like music, art is a highway to communication with the past. Must talk to Anna about the possibility.

There's not much to look forward to in going home. Same old, same old, but a possibility of improvement for Marsha. And if she improves, we both improve. Poor baby. My heart bleeds for her.

Anna returned with food and they ate leisurely, Marsha propped up on the bed with Jack sitting beside her, wielding the soup spoon.

They talked. Anna agreed the art is the work of patients, although she didn't know how much it meant in relating to past, present, or future. "If there were another day at the Oyam, or if we come back for the one-year follow-up study, we must remember to ask. I forgot to inquire–too busy trying to figure it out for myself earlier and then big distractions today."

They talked more. Jack had liked the story of the Alzheimer's patient who believed he still taught a physics class and all the others at the daycare facility were his students. He complained constantly that they didn't do their homework and never turned in their assignments. When a staff member started giving him a stack of papers with random markings on them, he loved it.

Spent hours correcting these papers and talking about what they meant.

Anna like the story of the woman who had worked on a cruise ship for a few years long ago. In her facility, she felt in charge of everyone's recreational activities. She'd offer to assist in planning a day of interesting things to see or to do. She asked each person how he or she was enjoying the day and what each signed up for the next day.

Both of these were positive attitudes shown in Alzheimer's patients. Other stories related negative behaviors, erratic movements, outbursts, or like Marsha, climbing into a shell and living there all the time.

Who knows? Anna and I could be victims too. It's like an evil epidemic. Thank God for places like this that strive to find cause, prevention, care, and cure. He'd like to live to see good answers come on the scene.

Marsha and Karl were bathed, shampooed, and dressed for night by eight o'clock. "Now it's our time. Please hold me." Anna looked imploringly at Jack. "I feel I betrayed you today by repeating what Kyalene told me. Can you forgive me?"

"Of course. You acted wisely. You were trying to save Marsha's life, for God's sake. Nothing to take any blame for."

"Thank you Jack. I needed to hear that. I felt so guilty."

"Tonight is ours. I know how I want to spend it."

"I'll spend it in the same place, spend everything I have." Anna laughed, "To think that I had this plan for us to sightsee all around. Sightseeing can't compete with lovemaking as a pleasurable activity."

"Right. I just want to be with you and without anyone else or anything else. There are three great things in my life–you, you, and you." He held her. "Want to dance?"

"Turn on the music. Remember dancing is making love to music. If we make love to music it must be dancing. Let's dance. The theme song should be 'I Love Being Loved by You'."

"A good one. I hear Ronnie Milsap singing 'What a Difference You Made in My Life'. He's singing my song to you. I thank you so much Anna. I am different because of you. You brought me to life and made my life worth living."

"Should we give The Clinic credit for a pair of miracle cures? It happened on their turf."

"Why not? They're famous for fixing what ails folks. Wouldn't have happened were we not here—together." Jack rubbed his face in her hair.

The two-way emotional support and physical activity served as effective medicine for the "downs" of this day. They fell asleep in each other's arms, exhausted and happy.

14 Anna

Anna lay in their bed, awake in the darkened room, enjoying the feel of Jack's warm body wrapped around hers. She gently extricated herself from his embrace so she could roll over toward the bedside table. The red digital numbers on the bedside clock read 4:10. The alarm wouldn't go off for over an hour.

Jack breathed the regular, quiet breaths of peaceful sleep beside her. How dear this man had become in such a short time. Anna moved closer again, settling on Jack's arm and reaching across his chest to be as close as possible yet not disturb him. She stroked his skin lightly, thinking about the feel of skin. This must be why silk is considered such a luxurious fabric; the feel of silk is like human skin.

Jack stirred slightly, then wrapped his other arm around her, not breaking the rhythm of his breathing. How wonderful to be held like this, thought Anna. I didn't know how much I needed loving.

Jack and Marsha's plane wouldn't leave until 9:00 this morning, but they needed to report in at the airport by 7:30 to turn in the rental car and check in at the airline. With Marsha as a passenger using a wheelchair, there would be early boarding for them. At this small airport, there should be plenty of time.

They would breakfast at the motel, Jack and Marsha would be off to California, and Anna might never see Jack again. Tears came unbidden to her eyes. Tomorrow might be the end. The end of this wonderful week and the end of knowing Jack. What are the chances we would both return with Marsha and Karl for the one-year follow-up visit to Oyam? With Karl and Marsha both worsening, who could know what would happen in a year. One or the other might be unable to travel. Without The Clinic study, the odds against their seeing each other again approached infinity.

Jack gone! Anna felt panic. How could they part so soon? They had just found each other. Almost a one-night stand. She had to smile—perhaps seniors needed several nights to be the equivalent of a one-night.

Sobering, she tensed. This parting could *not* be happening. She hugged Jack, still careful not to awaken him, but needing to capture every moment as intensely as possible. Anna needed him. She wanted to be with him forever. She, the strong, independent one, now so dependent on one man, this one man. What was happening to her? How could she go back to her life before this week at The Clinic? Her tears were now wetting the pillow.

What choice was there—she knew no alternative existed. Forget it for now, she told herself; just enjoy these last chips of time and don't think ahead. There would be plenty of time to ponder all that had happened in the next days, weeks, and months. She knew she would remember details of this week so long as she lived.

Whispering, Anna said, "I'll never forget you or anything about this week. I'll be thinking of you with every breath I take for the rest of my life."

Jack moved, pulling his arm out from under her head and shoulder and turning her around, facing away from him. They drew into their now-customary sleeping position. His arms around her made her feel snug and protected from anything the world might throw in her path. One of his hands cupped her lower breast, as usual. It seemed they had been together half a century, not this little shred torn from real time. He stirred again and Anna could feel that he was aroused.

"What time is it?" Jack muttered in a sleep-filled voice. Anna told him it was 5:00 and the alarm was set to go off in 20 minutes.

"Shut it off, please, " Jack loosened his hold, she reached for the clock, clicked it off, and turned to face Jack in bed. "One more time, Anna, let's make one more memory to nourish us when we're apart."

As Anna arose to enter the bathroom, she sang to Jack, "Other nights and other days will find us gone our separate ways, but we will have these moments to remember." She stopped, looking contemplative, "That should be our theme song for this week." Karl and Marsha lost their memories. A mind is a terrible thing to lose. This week we built memories, new and wonderful memories, as varied as a trip to an exotic foreign land."

They made love without hurry, enjoying every touch, every kiss, every moment of the act. Fulfilled, they clung to each other. Anna's tears welled with emotion as she thought, "I love this man, I lust for this man. Love and lust go hand in hand. I used to think they were opposites."

"Jack, there is so much I want to say. Words, even those in songs, can't express the deep feeling I have for you and the sadness at being away from you."

"I know, I know," Jack murmured in her ear, "You know I have exactly the same feelings. Farewell songs abound. The pain of parting set to music. Let's see, there's 'after you've gone and left me crying, after you've gone, there's no denying, you'll feel blue, you'll feel sad, we've lost the bestest thing we've ever had'."

"That's good Jack , and true. What else can we think of? How about 'Remember Me, I'm the One Who Loves You'?"

"Good one too. There must be a thousand more. We'll think of them and keep them 'Among Our Souvenirs'."

"My farewell song to you is Dolly Parton's 'I Will Always Love You'. Dearest Jack, that says it for me."

"We'll make that a duet. We are mates, soul mates and music mates too." They gripped each other as though letting go meant certain, instant death.

After a quiet few moments, Jack said, "Got to get going. Who's first in the shower or shall we share it?" He seemed awake and energetic. Anna couldn't decline the offer of showering together. She would leap at any and all opportunities to be as close to him as possible.

Pink and damp after the shower, Anna offered to get breakfast from the motel eating area and bring it to the room. Jack agreed that was a good idea, and came with her to carry one of the trays.

Marsha was awake and ready to get up when the food filled the small table in the room. Jack turned on the television to check the weather for Minnesota and for California. Karl slept soundly in spite of the talking and the TV. As always, Marsha obediently opened her mouth for each spoonful of oatmeal Jack fed her.

"I'll clear everything away later. Don't bother with picking up," Anna advised Jack. Anna watched Jack pack his razor in his toiletries bag, stow it in his large suitcase, and close it. She smiled up at him, "I like it that you always think of shaving before kissing me. That's a level of consideration I have never encountered and I love it. You've spoiled me."

"If I'm given credit for anything you like, I'll gladly take it. Now let's see if we have separated the Rutherford things from the Schmidt things. It's a little crazy how we've become so entwined—I mean our possessions, not just the two new couplings the four of us have fashioned. Hey, I've got a name for this week. What do you think of Re-Pairing at The Clinic?"

"Jack, that's clever. It says it all in four words. Maybe you could write a song under that title."

They looked carefully through both rooms, assuring nothing was left in the one Jack would check out of and nothing of theirs was left among Anna and Karl's things. Jack put his arms around Anna as they stood in the center of the room, "Anna, the only thing I left here is my heart. I know it is in safe keeping with you. We must keep in touch. I couldn't go on without having you in my life. We'll call when we can. We'll email, we'll use Skype, whatever, but we must keep in touch. Will you promise?" There were tears in Jack's eyes.

"Oh, yes," Anna breathed deeply and kissed him, "I want that as much as you do. I promise to keep in touch. I have your home and email address, your home and cell phone numbers and you have mine, so we're equipped with all the communication tools. Please call me on my cell phone when you get home as we may not be back in Bemidji before you arrive in Thousand Oaks."

Jack said he would, then hurried to check out at the desk and stow their suitcases and Marsha's wheelchair in the car. Time seemed to speed up. Anna could feel that she was breathing rapidly, as though she were running a race. Karl slumbered on, so Anna walked out with Jack on his last trip to the car. Outside the room door, he kissed her again and murmured, "I love you" in her ear. Soon he was outside, Marsha slumped in the seat beside him, the motor running. Anna waved from the motel entrance.

Suddenly she wanted to run to him, to beg him to stay, or beg him to take her with him, or just beg to be kissed one more time. She knew she could do none of those things. She had no claim on him. They each had their "obligations" as he had put it, meaning their spouses and their marriages. Anna's family, society's expectations, and heaven knows how many other things could be under her umbrella of "obligations".

As Jack pulled the car away from the motel, tears suddenly cascaded down Anna's cheeks. She felt deserted, alone, frightened of the future, frightened by the power of her emotions, and as out of control as she had been when they had first met under that cafeteria table.

"This isn't like me. I must go back to being the ME I was before this week," Anna said aloud. She picked up another cup of coffee on the way back to her room. There she sipped her drink and watched Karl in sleep. His beautiful silver, wavy hair mussed from turning his head on the pillow. Just looking at him, Anna thought of music as though it were an equation, Karl equals music plus singing. She wondered how many farewell songs he knew.

She tried to remember a song that she had heard him sing with Jenny Peters, How did it go? A line came to Anna: "Our love affair is a wondrous thing that we'll rejoice in remembering." The tears flowed afresh.

Agonizingly she prodded these thoughts out of her mind, saving the pondering time for when she would be back home in Bemidji with Karl. Alone with these young memories that would never age. There would be songs to burnish the memories. So many songs. The songs would remember.

Afterword

Charlie Marks, good friend and gifted surgeon, also enjoyed fishing. His granddaughter wrote the following poem, which was used at final services for him. It seems a fitting end to this book as well.

Charlie's Release

by Marie Kutz-Marks

In a vine-bathed swamp, deep
in the mind, he greets the ribbons
of carp as they skirt his small boat,
sun peeking through the hanging moss.

A disease of forgotten names fleshes
into forgotten faces as memory grays,
unraveling the smooth tufts above
his spotted ears. Years of color dim.

Charlie caresses the still water
with two long and knobby fingers,
knowing the rhythm of this place.
The sky breathes into his quivering lip.

Shaking wide-eyed through the house
he cannot remember how to cry
and loses himself among the family:
too many strangers with neon voices.
A cavernous owl hole creaks softly,
stretching its bark-encrusted cavity,
as the mother-branches above reach
for his boat across the gentle wake.

Charlie's wife watches from the bedside
as his eyes swim fast under their lids.
Today she says, "Charlie...it's alright."
"Yes," he thinks, "a good day for fishing."